WE ARE WINNING

Positive Emotion!

I CHOOSE TO FIGHT

I CHOOSE TO FIGHT

Tom Harper's
Courageous Victory
Over Cancer

Randy Harper and Tom Harper

Prentice-Hall, Inc.
Englewood Cliffs, New Jersey

Prentice-Hall, Inc. Englewood Cliffs, N.J.
Prentice-Hall International, Inc., *London*
Prentice-Hall of Australia, Pty. Ltd., *Sydney*
Prentice-Hall Canada, Inc., *Toronto*
Prentice-Hall of India Private Ltd., *New Delhi*
Prentice-Hall of Japan, Inc., *Tokyo*
Prentice-Hall of Southeast Asia Pte. Ltd., *Singapore*
Whitehall Books, Ltd., Wellington, *New Zealand*
Editora Prentice-Hall do Brasil Ltda., *Rio de Janeiro*

© 1984 *by*
RTJ COMPANY, INC.

Library of Congress Cataloging in Publication Data

Harper, Randy.
  I choose to fight.

  1. Harper, Tom, 1953-   . 2. Cancer--Patients--
United States--Biography. I. Harper, Tom, 1953-
II. Title.
RC265.6.H37H37   1984   362.1'96994   [B]   84-2040
ISBN 0-13-448911-X

Printed in the United States of America

Dedicated to

Our parents,
Jackson and Dorothy Harper

and to

Vice Admiral William P. Mack, USN (retired)
Superintendent, United States Naval Academy
1972–1975
"Tom's got a chance."

Vice Admiral Kinnard McKee, USN
Superintendent, United States Naval Academy
1975–1978
"Tom Harper can stay here until he either dies
or graduates."

PROLOGUE

When Tom and I had finished working on *I Choose to Fight*, it became clear to me that, while an important part of the story is the fact that my brother recovered successfully from cancer, a better thing to remember is that he chose to fight with every fiber of his body, regardless of the consequences. A commitment to fight cannot guarantee that a cancer patient will beat this disease, but a positive attitude is nevertheless of considerable therapeutic value.

There is a biblical legend about the pool of Bethesda, where an angel came once a year to ripple the waters. Anyone who was in the water when this happened was cured of all their ailments. A crippled, paralyzed man lay for years by the pool, waiting for someone to put him in the water, but people were so anxious to get in themselves that every year he was passed by, and so he remained, forgotten, alone on the shore. Jesus came one day and said to him, "Do you want to walk?" The poor man, of course, answered, "Yes." "Well," Jesus replied, "get up, then, and walk!" Upon hearing this, the man thought for a moment, then rolled off his pallet and walked away.

The point of this story is not to talk about miracles, but rather to point out that it was the man's own faith that cured him, not the waters of Bethesda. That faith is the equivalent of Tom Harper's commitment to fight cancer, to do something, anything, in order to survive. He could very well have died from testicular cancer, but he would have died fighting, never giving an inch. What happened to my brother can happen to anyone. His appreciation of life is the most important part of his story, and sharing this appreciation represents, perhaps, the best contribution that either one of us will ever make.

Randy Harper

INTRODUCTION

Cancer is an equal opportunity killer, and it chose me. I was admitted to the Bethesda Naval Hospital on Friday, September 28, 1973, with a baseball-sized, malignant tumor in my left testicle. I was a 19-year-old Naval Academy midshipman and a good athlete and football player, but cancer was crawling inside my body.

I lost my hair, my muscle tone, and my strength. I suffered severe acne, constant diarrhea, and daily vomiting, losing 50 pounds within four weeks. My mouth was filled with sores, my fingernails fell off, and my eyesight was often blurry and distorted. I couldn't remember anything at times. The radiation and drug treatments were powerful in a terrible sort of way, but the nights spent with other dying patients, the depression, and the lonely anguish—these were far worse. I was given 90 days to live, never to make it out of the hospital, much less to be processed out of the Naval Academy as medically unfit. If the disease didn't kill me, the treatment certainly would.

I never believed that prognosis. I made a commitment to survive, to be involved, to play football again, and to be a commissioned Naval Academy graduate.

I had to do everything expected of any healthy midshipman while fighting the disease, and thus I had no choice but to be as positive as I could, to do whatever it took to recover. Anything. Some people rightly felt they were looking at a dead man, but I knew differently. There was the motivation and support of the U.S. Naval Academy, my family, good doctors and nurses, and the grace of God.

CHAPTER ONE

Dear Tom,

    I understand from the coaching staff at the Naval Academy that you are an outstanding athlete who has one more year of high school ahead of you. I know that it is early for you to think of the institution that you will attend to further your education, but, if I may, I would like to advise you to give the Naval Academy a great deal of consideration. I had the good fortune to graduate from Navy, and if I had it to do over again, I wouldn't change one thing or one part of my decision. The Naval Academy is a tremendous place. All I ask is that you thoroughly investigate it.

    Best wishes in the coming football season.

Sincerely,
Roger Staubach

    The sun always seems to set slowly along the Chesapeake Bay and around Annapolis, through changing seasons and the humid winds of summer, when time stands still along the Severn River.

    Annapolis is 30 miles or so east of the nation's capital and is a city of unique combinations, with buildings of Early American architecture and cosmopolitan tradition. Eighteenth-century homes still stand, trimmed by gently rising, narrow streets and brick sidewalks, garnished with the window dressings of quaint shops up from the fish market and the docks below. The waterfront location by the Severn River and Chesapeake Bay, together with rich heritage and the splendid old structure of the town, makes it a pleasant and special city.

The Naval Academy's rock sea wall along the eastern flank holds back the bay, the sound of harbor bells complementing the Academy's granite gray buildings set back from the water's edge. The landscape behind the perimeter walls, with soft green turf, large trees, and several colors of flowers, serves as a perfect aerial border. The Academy is a natural to Annapolis, dating back to 1826 when the Maryland General Assembly solicited the federal government for a study of Annapolis as a suitable locale for a naval school.

The chapel is the centerpiece of the Academy Yard, covering the ground like a large stone cross under a weathered copper dome, opening with huge bronze doors that proclaim in Latin, "Not for self, but for country." A small hospital sits on top of what was once known as Strawberry Hill, the residence of the last British colonial governor, overlooking athletic fields and the river. Quiet, stately, three-story homes along Upshur Road, quarters for senior Academy staff officers, ring the Worden Parade Field. The large gazebo bandstand on the east side of the field is visible from their front porches, where cannon smoke from festivities would sometimes wisp by with a change in the wind. Two years after getting that letter from Roger Staubach, I was sworn in as a midshipman along with 1300 other young men, as we assembled on July 7, 1973, in the vast courtyard of the Academy's only dormitory, Bancroft Hall.

My new platoon had gathered earlier for the march to the swearing-in ceremony on a red-tiled deck somewhere in the maze of Bancroft. It became a hot, muggy afternoon, and the clippings of my fresh haircut rolled between my neck and the white collar of my uniform as we marched outside. Most of us wore ill-fitting, sloppy new uniforms, crewcuts bobbing in and out of baggy garments, a little book entitled *Reef Points* stuck in everybody's pocket. I had spent the year before at the Naval Academy Prep School (NAPS), and my Marine instructor there, Captain Ralph Sinke, would have been visibly upset by this display.

Senior midshipmen marched out smartly from Bancroft Hall's rotunda to mark the beginning of formalities. There were some short remarks by various admirals and navy captains and interludes of band music, and soon I found myself standing with everybody else to recite the induction oath. I remember thinking that if I was going to change my mind I'd better do it quickly. But I repeated the oath completely and rendered a salute, along with all my classmates, as the national anthem was played.

I was recruited by several schools, including Navy, during my last two years of high school in San Bruno, California. I didn't honestly know if I could play major college football, or even if I wanted to, and the Naval Academy offered me a chance to play football and receive a quality education. My older brother had gone there, but my family didn't really have a military background, and I wasn't that iron-disciplined a person. I, like many 18-year-olds, didn't know exactly what I wanted to do right after high school. I liked everything I saw and heard about the Naval Academy, from the uniforms to the parades, from tradition to patriotism. It seemed to offer a sense of direction, but I was like most new midshipmen, because there was no single, specific reason why I wanted to be one. I knew however, what I would be when I graduated—a Naval Officer—and many of my high school friends had no idea of where they might end up out of college. I would have nothing to give up—a scholarship, or grant-in-aid—if I couldn't play college football. I would still be a midshipman. The education, the chance to learn discipline, the regimented schedule and certainly, the security, if I measured up—all these things appealed to me. The Naval Academy seemed to be the best way to prepare for the future, even if I didn't make the Navy my career. Many of my friends were waiting to make up their minds about what they would do, which for them was probably the right thing. I would give up a lot of personal freedom, for awhile anyway, but I had the opportunity to be a part of something unique. I was eighteen years old, and there was plenty of time.

I wasn't prepared academically for Annapolis, so when I was offered the opportunity to go to the Naval Academy's Prep School, I took it. I had to see what I could do, and I could still play for any other major school if I changed my mind. I put a lot of effort into NAPS, studies, football, and especially weight lifting. Captain Sinke had told me he thought I was the only NAPS football player who could make the Navy varsity as a freshman. After months of all that, I guess I was psyched to prove, not only to myself but to everybody else, that I could play major college football and carry a full load of classes.

We had gone through a rather routine process during check-in as midshipman candidates. There had been no yelling, no running, no squaring corners; everything was rather subdued. Registration, gear draw, room assignment—these were small hassles at first, but so far there had been none of the horror stories we'd been fed at NAPS. The main priority seemed to be stenciling our day-old midshipman identification numbers onto our new clothes. Lunch earlier in the mess hall had been our first real plebe occasion, but it was uneventful, and I was beginning to wonder if everything I'd heard about "Plebe Summer" was true.

I spotted another fellow NAPSter, Dan Ashby, after the induction, and we decided to walk casually back to our rooms. "What are you two idiots doing? Why are you walking? Run, run, run! Get going, plebe! Move it, Mister! Get your ass in gear, plebe!" First classmen came out of nowhere, screaming, "Double time! Double time! Double time!" Ashby and I momentarily froze in our tracks, startled by this sheer madness that came without warning. We started to run together, our chins tucked in and fists pumping madly at our sides, following an imaginary line down the middle of a long hall somewhere in "Mother B" (Bancroft Hall). Dan had to go down a different corridor toward his room, and I yelled at him, "Well, I guess it's started!"

"Yep!"

I continued straight ahead and didn't see Ashby again for two months.

There were no more leisurely meals, and dinner that night was quite different. Straight back in our chairs, we plebes sat, no elbows on the table and feet perfectly on the floor, hearing with chins tucked in about how to speak like a plebe, how to pass food like a plebe, what to memorize like a plebe, how to dress like a plebe, how to speak to an upper-classman like a plebe, how to go to the bathroom like a plebe. The rest of the night was more of the same—marching, folding clothes, sorting things out, sitting in a hot and sweaty group listening to our revered squad leaders lecture on a variety of subjects. The lights went out much too early, but my roommate and I stayed up an extra two hours, studying and memorizing a little blue book full of Navy facts and figures, the *Reef Points* bible, under my miniature flashlight.

The schedule was intense, and we were running from dawn to past taps. There were tests and tests and more tests, plebe "rates" to memorize, physical and mental harassment periods called come-arounds every day, memory drills, and, foremost, a cultivated fear of the upperclassmen. Ten minutes before each of the three formations of the day, I was in front of my upperclassman's door, pounding three times and yelling, "Midshipman Fourth Class Harper, Sir! Permission to come aboard, Sir!"

"Enter, Plebe."

Once allowed access into those hallowed chambers, I was at stiff attention, looking straight ahead, afraid to move a muscle, ready to recite answers to any series of rates that could be demanded. How many days till Army? How many days till Christmas leave? How many days till I graduate? How many days till the Second Class Ring Dance? What are the movies in town? Discuss three articles from the sports page. What are the tactical jets in the Navy inventory? What are the ships in a carrier task force? What's the dinner menu? Breakfast? Lunch? Who's the officer of the watch?

There were always new questions when the old ones ran out, and more verbal abuse during meals, when we had to serve the upperclassmen. "Why did you let my glass become half empty?" or "Why did you fill my glass up again, you idiot?" We even sneaked out at night to use the lavatory down the hall, lest we be seen by the feared upperclassmen. I never used the open urinal, always availing myself of the privacy and relative safety of the enclosed commodes. Obviously, you couldn't win.

Chow calls were races against the clock, as we shouted

for ten minutes, generally in one-minute intervals, before formation: the menu for the upcoming meal, personnel on watch, the movies in town, and whatever else the upperclassmen wanted to hear, usually from a point in Bancroft Hall farthest away from where our company would be assembled. The race to formation after the last call was sheer panic, and I had but one single purpose in life then—to get to formation on time. Even that brought mixed consequences, because invariably I'd get there in time, but dripping with sweat, with a scuffed shoe or some other uniform aberration. There was always something they could get you on. Uniform races were no fun, either. The races involved constant changes of dress, anywhere from full formal dress to running gear to the uniform of the day and back again. These maneuvers usually destroyed both the manicured look of the garments and the neatness of the clothes lockers, which we all had so painstakingly arranged.

"PEP" was every day—5:15 A.M. physical exercise drills that often began only a couple of hours after I went to bed. We had ten minutes after PEP to shower, shave, dress in a clean uniform, and be in formation ready to march to breakfast. It was day-to-day survival.

Football practice finally arrived in late August. George Welsh was beginning his first year as Navy's head football coach, in charge of a program that had fallen on hard times in recent years. He had a tough job ahead, and a break-even season would be a marked improvement for a team that hadn't enjoyed a winning season since my older brother's plebe year in 1967. The glory days of Staubach and company were a long time ago, and poor seasons didn't help the recruiting challenge, already difficult because of lucrative professional contracts and the Academy's five-year service commitment. Coach Welsh had been an assistant coach at Penn State for the previous ten years, but he certainly was familiar with the Academy and Navy football. He was a 1956 Annapolis graduate, an All-American quarterback, and he played in the 1956 Sugar Bowl. He was a quiet and reserved man, very professional, and unbelievably intense on the playing field.

There was an increased level of competition at Navy, much more than what I had experienced in high school, but I'd been prepared well at NAPS and made steady progress during the summer football drills. Navy Commander Earle Smith, who also played for the Academy in the 1950s, was the tight end coach and took a liking to me, passing on comments about my "good hands," "quickness," and "uncanny reactions" to Coach Welsh.

The plebes on the football team were invited near the end of the summer to a formal dinner at the superintendent's quarters. The athletic director told me then that I'd made the travel squad, but that good news was marked by our group embarrassment of not knowing what to do with the dainty finger bowls and small towels presented to us after the meal. We were big, new college football players, in peak condition, ready for the start of the season, but no one knew what to do with the little bowls. The superintendent, Admiral William P. Mack, had to give us all a lesson in finger bowl etiquette. "OK, fellows, this is how you do it," he said as, in a manly way, he delicately patted each of his fingers dry. It was an awkward moment but fortunately soon forgotten, because as soon as we got back to our rooms there would be something new and different from the upperclassmen to worry about.

I first noticed it while I was taking a shower, halfway through Plebe Summer. I didn't want to say anything; I couldn't afford the reputation that I couldn't hack it, and I thought the symptom, though painful, was similar to other plebe hurts such as pulled muscles or tendonitis. My left testicle was the size of a small fist. Several football players had mentioned that I ought to have it checked out, but I didn't want to consult a doctor. It was sure to go away and, besides, I had established somewhat of a routine, as most every plebe had, of dealing with Plebe Summer. I didn't want any disruptions.

Soon, however, there were many summer evenings when I couldn't sleep because of this pain, enduring it while studying plebe rates, looking out the window at the blackness of the night. Sometimes I'd manage only two or three hours of rest, doubled up in pain, curled up so as not to disturb my roommates or embarrass myself. I began to feel bad everywhere. I didn't know what was causing the pain, and even though there were excruciating shots through my abdomen and up my spine, I never thought it was truly serious. It just wouldn't go away, and I didn't feel as quick or as confident as I needed to be. I worried about it, but only when I actually hurt; when it momentarily went away, I forgot about it, because being a plebe was worry enough.

Finally, it hurt so much that I had to complain to the Navy trainer, who sent me to see Dr. Marty Eichelberger and Dr. Bill Clancy, the team doctors.

"Have you been screwing around, Tom?" Dr. Clancy asked.

"Bill, he's just a plebe. He's been here all summer," Dr. Eichelberger replied, before I could answer.

"Oh, yeah," Dr. Clancy said, chuckling. "Sorry, Tom."

I mentioned abdominal pains to Dr. Eichelberger for the next few days, as did several other players. The muggy Annapolis summer lent itself quite well to dehydration, and that, combined with epididymis, a condition of sperm blockage, was Dr. Eichelberger's initial diagnosis. Utilization of the proper prescription usually cleared up the matter in about ten days, and sick bay passed the right dosage along to me. I didn't tell anyone that for almost two weeks I hadn't had a bowel movement.

Though at times I thought the ritual would never end, it was soon Parents' Weekend, marking almost the end of summer's humidity, with the conclusion of our summer "fun." It was my parents' second summer visit after seven years to the Academy, and I was happy to see Mom and Dad. I had been through something and enjoyed sharing it with them. I have two brothers and five sisters, and although I wasn't really homesick, I thought about everybody often, wondering what they were all up to. I was tied up with football practice at the start of the weekend, and I twisted my ankle on the astroturf while running a pass play. My weekend schedule had to change, since I had to have whirlpool treatments, but my parents and I managed to tour the Academy grounds, though somewhat hesitantly. As we sat by the Tecumseh statue, I told Mom, "My stomach and side are killing me." It had to be an ordinary football contact.

Coach Welsh gave us Saturday afternoon off, but I had to undergo whirlpool therapy again, and my parents met me at sick bay that evening where I was elevating my ankle. I didn't mention the pain in my testicle or its growing size, and after they left I searched the quiet and deserted sick bay for something to ease my stomach. My ankle felt fine in comparison, and I didn't want to go into any lengthy ritual about it with the corpsman on duty. I found two large, full bottles of Pepto Bismol in a medicine cabinet and drank both of them. I felt bad enough as it was, being laid up in sick bay after my parents had flown out all the way from California.

September brought academics and a complete change of routine—study, study, study, staying up late at night, concentrating one minute on calculus, history, or chemistry and the next on duties for my squad leader or some other upperclassman.

My "Blue Book," the play book of the varsity football team, provided a unique way around the rigors of plebe year. It was simple—carry one, and no one bothered you. Especially when I wore a name tag without my class year on it. Most of the upperclassmen were not aware yet of the new NCAA rule that allowed freshmen to play varsity football. With a Blue Book, the upperclassmen thought I was one of them. I was lucky they didn't figure it out too soon.

Academics emphasized engineering, math, chemistry, and physics, but I parlayed the study of formulas and equations into such plebe rates as, "How's the cow?"

"Sir! She walks, she talks, she's full of chalk! The lacteal fluid extracted from the female of the bovine species is highly proficient to the 77th degree! Sir!"

This was meant to tell people how many glasses of milk were left in the blue Academy-crested cartons on the mess hall table.

"Why didn't you call me *Sir*?"

"Sir, Sir is a subservient word surviving from the surly

days in old Serbia when certain serfs, too ignorant to remember their lords' names, yet too servile to blaspheme them, circumvented the situation by surrogating the subservient word, Sir, by which I now belatedly address a certain senior cirriped, who correctly surmised that I was syrupy enough to say Sir after every word I said, Sir!"

"What time is it? Who's Horsecan Harry? The laws of the Navy? Man overboard drill! Mission of USNA. Chow call!"

And on and on and on. Somehow, though, it became easier to memorize things and organize my thoughts and my time.

I decided that nothing was going to stop me from playing football. My stomach cramps and swollen testicle were scary whenever the pain was bad, but I did my best to ignore it. I couldn't lose the opportunity to play, and whatever was wrong surely would go away. I continued taking the pills Dr. Eichelberger gave me, and the medication eased the discomfort a little.

Our first contest of the season was an away game against VMI, the Virginia Military Institute. Their stadium looked high-schoolish from the bus, but I lost any negative feelings when I put on my game uniform for the first time. The blue jersey and gold pants, the glint of my helmet—this was the beginning! Billy Smyth, a senior, was the starting tight end, and he'd confided to Al Glenny, our starting quarterback, that I'd be pressing him for the starting position as soon as my ankle healed completely.

Coach Welsh jolted me from the bench late in the fourth quarter, shouting, "Tommy Harper, tight end delay!"

I was wide open, it was a sure touchdown, but our second-string quarterback didn't see me as he ran around end for 14 yards. I took out my frustration by leveling a VMI defensive back with a body block.

The next week brought Penn State to Annapolis, and, as usual, Joe Paterno had his Nittany Lions nationally ranked. I didn't play a down in the Penn State game, Navy serving as fodder for the Nittany Lions' relentless advance in the polls. My closest point of contact came when I helped John Cappelletti, the Heisman Trophy winner that year, up from the sidelines after a rare tackle by our defense.

I didn't worry about my testicle symptoms or the pain as the month went on, because I was too busy to remember the day before, much less the admonitions of Dr. Eichelberger. It was time to get ready to play Michigan, our third game of the season, and after the practice week before playing the Wolverines, I was the number two tight end. Commander Smith told me to expect plenty of playing time, and I was definitely up. My ankle had healed, and our starting tight end was spending a lot of time practicing a new position with the defensive backs. I hoped to be starting by the second half of the Michigan game.

I concentrated hard on studies that week to avoid being overanxious about the game and my weekend plans with Susie McElroy, the sister of a close NAPS friend whose family lived near the Michigan campus. I spent several hours in the library, researching topics and sources for term papers, reading about famous men from history. It seemed to me that whatever the subconscious was, it could guarantee failure as easily as success, and this thought was reinforced by the traits of these historical and successful leaders. I had my best practices during the preparation for Michigan, convinced that I could eliminate the testicular pain from my state of mind. During the first practice, I missed a few blocks, and Coach Welsh passed by, saying, "C'mon, Harper, do it right. You've done it before."

I became psyched because he noticed me—he knew who Tom Harper was, a six-foot-three, 225-pound tight end, and I was at my best from then on.

The pain began to subside as the Michigan game drew closer, and Dr. Eichelberger had a ready supply of pills whenever I ran low. The team doctors were taking good care of me, and I didn't want to tell them anything that would cause alarm. I ran into Dr. Clancy by the locker room stairs the Thursday before Ann Arbor, and he asked if my testicle had cleared up. He seemed surprised when I told him it hadn't.

"I'll check with Marty," he said, and I thought maybe they'd just change the prescription.

It seemed, however, for the first time to be abnormal to have such a large lump hanging from my groin, but I just concentrated that much harder on putting that feeling out of my mind. It was more important to play against the Michigan Wolverines. I was on the varsity, with a chance to be one of the first plebes ever to start on a Navy football team. I had always been healthy, always in excellent physical condition, the captain of my high school football and basketball teams, and I had played hurt many times before. The pain became deeper and more intense almost hourly, but I persuaded myself to ignore it. It would go away, and by that evening, September 27, 1973, I was ready.

It would be beautiful the next couple of days in Ann Arbor—what an atmosphere! The crisp fall air mixed with colors, more than 100,000 enthusiastic people in the stands, the wind whistling through the famous tunnel of the Michigan stadium, the tailgate parties and collegiate enthusiasm—all this combined with my dream of playing for Navy against the number one team in the nation. The tight end coach had been preparing me all week, and I knew I would play. I was ready to be Navy's best tight end, and nothing else mattered.

CHAPTER TWO

I awoke shortly after sunrise, the alarm clock making a dull sound, incessant and steady, the luminous face glowing in the early light. Daybreak was along the far horizon, and glimpses of sky were possible through the upper part of the room windows, the blinds making a tinkering, rustled, bell-like sound with the wind.

I weighed 225 pounds, my weight training and lifting paying off, and I couldn't remember being in better shape. My left testicle still hurt, but I tried not to think about it, hoping it would go away. It was too grotesque to look at. The new pills Dr. Eichelberger had prescribed the day before seemed to help—my stomach ache wasn't as bad, but I needed more before leaving for Michigan.

I went through the morning plebe ritual by the numbers—shaving, shining shoes, and going down the hall for a routine head call although it had been almost three weeks since I had any type of bowel movement. I left for breakfast a few minutes earlier than normal.

The mess hall was huge, and the food was great. I enjoyed being with teammates at the training tables. There were no upperclassmen to harass me, no regimented stories to tell, no reports to make, nothing to recite. You just ate.

Everyone in our room had chores to do—just in case an upperclassman or an officer made an inspection, although my roommates and I weren't bothered as much as our other classmates in the 31st Company. We were nestled in an obscure

sixth-wing shaft, away from most of the company upperclassmen in the eighth wing of Bancroft Hall. Packing my travel
bag for Michigan, I concealed civilian clothes beneath text-
books I had promised myself to study. My last task before
class was to empty half a can of Pledge by the doorway so that
the floor reflected light from the hall with a spit-shined luster.

First period was chemistry, and I sat next to fellow ex-
NAPSters Steve Scott and Steve Barnett. We talked about the
game with Michigan as much as the prof talked about con-
version factors for the next test. I told them I was hurting.
Second period was sea power, my last class of the day, because the football team was leaving for Ann Arbor in a few
hours, and varsity players were excused by midmorning.

I walked to the eighth-wing locker room after sea power
and was one of the first players there. My testicle hurt as I
changed into white gym shorts, and for some reason it
seemed harder and bigger, but Dr. Eichelberger had examined
me the day before and didn't say much about it. I slipped on a
gray t-shirt, cut off at the midsection, and went upstairs to see
the doctor, taking the steps three at a time.

Dr. Eichelberger, alone in his office, looked up just as I
entered the doorway and walked up to his desk.

"Hey, Doc, you know those pills you gave me? Well, I
think they really worked, but I ran out a couple of days ago,
and my testicle is starting to hurt again. Can I get some
more?"

During my last examination with him, he had squeezed
my left testicle and asked if it hurt. I thought I was getting
away with something by saying I didn't feel a thing.

I handed him the empty pill vial. Dr. Eichelberger, leaning back in his chair, glanced at the label and then leaned
forward and put the pill container on his desk pad. The chair
creaked and moaned, and he tapped his fingers for a few seconds on its arms, staring in the general direction of the paperwork that covered his desk, not wanting to tell me everything
he thought. He'd been the team doctor only a few months.

"Tom, I'd like you to see Dr. Phil Landry up at the Academy Hospital. I've talked to him, and he'd like to take a look at you. He's chief of general surgery for us. He's waiting for you. Why don't you go on up there? It won't take but a minute. I'll tell Coach Welsh if you're late, but if you hurry you shouldn't miss too much."

This surprised me.

"Who am I supposed to see?"

"Dr. Landry. He's a good doctor, and I think he can help us. What time does the bus leave today?"

"Right after the pep rally, right after lunch. Do you want me to check with you when I get back?"

"No. I'll see you on the field. Dr. Landry is waiting for you, so hot-foot it up there."

"OK, Doc. See you later."

Dr. Landry was a pleasant, chubby man in his fifties. He was a doctor who appeared busy—an authority—but I was immediately comfortable with him after he indicated that I should take a seat.

"How are you today?"

"Pretty good, Sir. Dr. Eichelberger sent me up here to see you."

"Yes, and I have your file right here."

He spent a few minutes looking through my medical jacket. I could see "Harper, Thomas Jackson 500589765" written in black felt marker on the side edge of the folder, which wasn't very thick, and I wondered what was in there besides my routine physicals and maybe comments about my sprained ankle.

"Tom, let's have a look," Landry said, closing the file and placing it back on the center of his desk. I stood up without saying anything, undoing the drawstring of my white work trousers, moving forward a few steps, and looking sheepishly at the doctor. I felt ridiculous. I hated these kind of examinations.

"Right here's fine. Just drop your shorts, and let's get this checked out."

I dropped my trousers and underwear to the tops of my

shoes, put my hands on my hips, and looked at the picture of
Navy ships lining the wall next to his desk.

"Relax, Tom," Landry kept saying as he felt and examined the testicle. We talked about putting everything off until
Monday, and Dr. Landry seemed inclined to let me play
against Michigan. I'd see a specialist after the weekend.

I was in and out of Dr. Landry's office within 30 minutes.
I was changing again when Dr. Eichelberger called me from
the upstairs railing that squared the opening between the two
floors of the locker room.

"Hey, Tom, come on up here a minute."

I looked at the clock on the wall down from my locker.
There was only 20 minutes of practice left, and I didn't want
to be bothered. Why couldn't these people just give me the
right medicine and leave me alone?

"Come on into the office." Eichelberger sounded serious,
so I begrudgingly jogged into his office. He was sitting on the
edge of his desk, his arms folded tightly, and his voice
sounded more concerned than I'd ever heard him before.

"Tom, first we're making arrangements for you to get to
the game. We will make sure you get there."

What's he talking about? I wondered. We're leaving for
the game in a couple of hours. Jesus Christ, I'm losing practice
time every time I listen to him.

"We're going to send you to the Bethesda Naval Hospital.
I've talked with Dr. Landry and Bill Clancy. You'll see a specialist in the urology clinic."

"What's urology? Dr. Landry said they'd see me again
Monday. I'm not going to Michigan?"

"We'll get you a commercial flight. Don't worry about
Michigan, Tom. I'll see that you get there."

Eichelberger was interfering with what had been a decent
day up till now. He was sincere, but nevertheless my plans
were in jeopardy.

"I'll get to the game, Doc?" I said, shaking my head
slowly up and down.

"We'll drive you over to Bethesda. Commander Schmidt,

the football team officer rep, will get you a ticket. You can fly out commercially and meet everybody up there."

I wasn't concerned about what could be wrong with me; I had to be finished at Bethesda in time to catch the commercial flight to Ann Arbor. Besides, I'd miss the first big road trip pep rally, 4000 midshipmen cheering us on in front of the Tecumseh statue. Coach Welsh had also missed me at practice.

"I've made some arrangements for a date up there, Doctor," I said, taking a pencil and a piece of paper from his desk and writing down names and telephone numbers.

"If Commander Schmidt gets me a late flight and the team gets there before I do, I'll need to let people know. Would you tell them or have Coach Welsh let them know when I'm supposed to get there? They're expecting me." I paused, gave him the paper, and said, "I'm supposed to play a lot in the game tomorrow."

Dr. Eichelberger had followed my progress up the depth chart and knew I was the number two tight end.

"It's almost time for noon meal, Tom. I'll have a driver take you to Bethesda after you eat."

I stood in front of the doctor's desk for a second, noticed him glance away, and almost asked if we could forget the whole affair.

We were 1–1 for the young season, having had an easy time with VMI, but after Penn State Coach Welsh knew considerable improvement was an understatement. The Michigan Wolverines would probably be our toughest contest of the year.

He was leaving the practice field when Marty Eichelberger approached.

"Coach Welsh?"

"What can I do for you, Doc?"

"Coach, I've had to send Tommy Harper up to Bethesda. He has a lump on his testicle that needs to be examined by the urologist there."

"Is it anything serious?"

"Yes, I'm afraid it is. He very possibly has a tumor. We've treated him with antibiotics for the past few days. Bill Clancy and I both examined him closely, along with Dr. Landry up on the hill. Tommy's been complaining of pain in the groin area. It doesn't look that good to me."

Eichelberger shook his head slowly, an urgency in his voice, never liking to tell Coach Welsh bad news about any of his players.

George knew immediately that it was serious—having to send me to Bethesda was all the indication he needed—but it was hard to imagine a healthy, 19-year-old athlete with this kind of problem. He didn't want to think about what could happen to me, or any other of his athletes in similar circumstances.

"Listen, Marty, be sure and keep me posted. Let me or one of the other coaches know as soon as you hear anything." He paused momentarily, then continued, "Do you think he'll be at Bethesda long?"

"It depends on the examination. If they take a biopsy, he'll be there at least a week, even if it's benign. If it's malignant . . ."

Dr. Eichelberger let the conversation drop. George Welsh knew what he was telling him.

The team doctor walked slowly back to the office he shared with Bill Clancy. It was a brisk fall day, and the high windows of the eighth-wing locker room were cracked open at topside, a crisp breeze helping to clear out the liniment smell. Skip Kaleta, the senior equipment manager, was standing by the stairway leading to the office.

"How are ya doing, Doc? Ready for your first trip?"

The doctor managed a smile.

"It should be a good time, Skip, for sure. I hope the boys are ready for a tough game."

He started up the stairs, but paused and turned back around.

"Say, Skip . . ."

"Yeah, Doc?"

"Ah . . . don't worry about Tommy Harper's gear. He won't be going with us."

"Is something wrong?"

"Yes, and we've had to send him to Bethesda. He . . . well, listen, Skip, I'll talk to you about it later."

Bill Clancy was in the small office, a simple room furnished with a desk, gray metal lockers, and two examination tables hidden under the bandages, tape, and other equipment used for lacerations and minor wounds.

"I got a driver for Tommy Harper, Bill. He'll take him to Bethesda right after lunch."

Clancy nodded in response and then replied, "Okay. Jesus, it's too bad. I hope Leftwich up there can give us some good word."

Dr. Eichelberger leaned against the green exam table by the door and reviewed my case. Just a month before, I'd come to them after talking with Red Romo, the head trainer, about abdominal pain—not uncommon with players who suffered heat stroke or exhaustion. Several of us had experienced cramps throughout the long, hot summer practices. The antibiotics had relieved some of my testicular pain, and they'd both seen me perform in practice, where I'd appeared to be in normal health. I hadn't been complaining too much, but my left testicle was hard, ugly, and large.

I spoke with some other football players about the hospital, and, while they offered words of encouragement, I felt uneasy. I was scared but didn't know what I was scared about. I didn't enjoy eating lunch like I usually did, and Randy Mikal, the senior starting offensive right guard, noticed I wasn't my usual self. He asked, "Hey, Tom, what's up?"

I filled Mikal in on what had happened, especially to my weekend plans. Mikal, feeling my uneasiness, put his hand on my shoulder and said, "Hey, don't worry about it. Everything will work out, Tommy."

I had butterflies in my stomach, and it wasn't even game time.

After lunch, I packed quickly for Bethesda—service dress blues and my overnight bag were all that I needed. It was the first time I had worn the blue Navy suit, so I studied the jacket carefully. The trousers fit snugly, and I found a use for the cuff links with the Academy crest design, putting a dimple in my tie and giving my shirt an extra tuck, even though the crease would be covered by my jacket. I didn't know how to rig the coat. Which way do the anchors go? What about the ribbons? Do they go one inch or two inches over the pocket? Are they straight or at an angle? I didn't dare go outside with everything positioned the wrong way. Luckily, a friendly upperclassman who occasionally dropped in was passing by, and he helped me put everything on correctly.

I felt sharp and squared away in my new uniform, and Dr. Eichelberger looked impressed when he met me in the parking lot, where a corpsman waited in a gray Navy station wagon.

"Midshipman Harper, you look terrific! I'm impressed! Do you look like a stud, or what?"

He saluted me, and the only thing I could think to say was, "Yes, sir. Thank you," grinning, surprised that a lieutenant would greet a plebe that way.

"You have my tickets? You did talk to Coach Welsh about my friends in Michigan?"

"Sure did, Tom. Bob . . . er . . . Commander Schmidt will get you squared away. We're taking care of it."

Eichelberger opened the right front door of the station wagon. "You look good. You'll knock 'em dead."

He clasped my shoulder and extended a firm handshake, and I didn't realize then that he was reinforcing my self-image for what could eventually happen. It was important to him not to even hint yet of what could be wrong, at least until a qualified diagnosis was available, owing to the outside chance that both his and Dr. Clancy's concern would be alleviated by a finding of something other than testicular cancer.

Eichelberger shut the door after I got in and stood there smiling. It seemed strange to me that I'd have to come back to the Academy for the commercial tickets, when the hospital was on the way to the airport. I didn't want to go to the hospital and didn't want another doctor looking at me. What would they find wrong? Whatever it was had better not screw up my plans.

The pep rally was starting as we drove through the gate and into a beautiful, vivid day, the countryside green and growing familiar. The drive reminded me of when I had visited the Academy during my senior year of high school with several other northern California recruits. The bus ride on Highway 50 then, as now, added a soothing touch, the rolling terrain bringing back memories of earlier grade school years when my family lived in North Carolina. Several red brick, two-story buildings sat back from the roadside, the white-pillared facades blending into lush vegetation and forest trees that spread all the way to the horizon. We passed the Mormon Tabernacle under construction and finally made it to the off-highway roads leading to Bethesda. I noticed the tall white building blocks away, on the outskirts of Chevy Chase just a few minutes from Georgetown. I first saw the sign as the driver pressed the left turn signal and turned off Wisconsin Avenue—"National Naval Medical Center." The gray station wagon eased up the long, half-circle entrance drive that enveloped several acres of manicured grass.

The main tower rose up more than 150 feet, with lower wings forming an architectural loop to the north and south, overlooking slow-rising steps flanked by evergreens. The national flag rolled with the quiet, lapping wind, the hospital a tall stone edifice outlined against the blue sky, sunlight reflecting through the car windows onto my black, spit-shined shoes. The driver stopped by a tall ship's mast that stood as a flagpole directly in line with the main entrance, and gave me directions to the urology clinic.

I didn't know anything about this hospital, other than vague recollections of presidents coming here, and though proud to be wearing my new service dress-blue uniform, I felt self-conscious because I'd left my hat in the back seat of the Navy car.

I entered a large, oversized, shiny foyer with four big marble pillars, somewhat darker and more grayish than the outside stone, commanded by railings guarding portraits of Navy surgeon generals. The hospital was noisy, with an air of urgency and medical mystique, and filled with that peculiar scent all hospitals seem to have. There were many serious-looking people carrying charts and clipboards, and I went past the emergency room, the pharmacy, and down narrow halls lined with outdated radiators and wide windows, the wall surface like bathroom ceramic tile.

The sign was simple enough—"Urology Clinic." I paused by the double doors, then pulled open the right one. I could see a receptionist seated at a large, circular platform.

"Hi, I'm Midshipman Harper."

She looked at me hesitantly, then seemed to remember something she had been told earlier.

"Midshipman Harper? Oh, yes. We've been expecting you. Why don't you have a seat, please?"

"Yes, Ma'am, thank you."

She smiled, adjusted her eyeglasses, and reached for the telephone.

It was less than a minute later when she said, "Right this way, Mr. Harper," gesturing toward Dr. Leftwich's office.

Dr. Frederick Leftwich hung up the phone as I came in. "Please have a seat. Relax. Take off your coat," he said, not standing up as he motioned me to give him the medical jacket I'd carried from the Academy. I leaned forward and gave him the file, draping my uniform blouse over my left arm. I could see Leftwich had some other notes already, and we sat silently for a few minutes, the doctor studying my file intently. He seemed to be an organized man, subdued, maybe tired, of average height and medium build, balding on top. He asked me about the symptoms and pain, and I told him about the nights without sleep during Plebe Summer, the swelling of my left testicle, and the pain in my abdomen.

"Was there anything else?"

"Well, Doctor, I've had trouble having any sort of bowel movement. The pain would subside if I doubled up and slept like a baby. My left testicle has been as hard as a rock, and it's a lot larger than my right one."

"I see. OK, Tom, let's go to the examination room and take a look."

Leftwich nodded in the direction over my right shoulder, and I took this as a signal to leave, remembering halfway out of his office that I was out of uniform. I stopped to put my coat back on, adjusting the cuffs as I went out.

The examination room was antiseptic, stark, with a white dressing curtain along one wall, the floor not carpeted and cold as I took off my clothes. Medical accoutrements were neatly placed on top of simple-looking equipment, and there was fresh paper on top of a padded table. There was only one chair. I felt like I was about to be violated, and for no good reason. I stripped down to my shorts, feeling awkward, sitting alone in this sterile room, my uniform hanging on the doorknob, and I hoped that no one other than Dr. Leftwich would open the door. I wanted everything to go quickly so that I could catch my flight to Michigan.

The examination was like the others, except that Leftwich had me lie on the table and probed around my groin and abdomen. I closed my eyes, breathed easily, and tried to relax.

"OK, I'm done for now," Leftwich said, and I sat up, pulling up my shorts and swinging my legs back over the table. Leftwich was washing his hands in a small sink that I hadn't noticed before.

"Why don't you go over to x ray. Use the green robe." He nodded again, this time toward the dressing curtain, where a green gown hung over the top of the frame.

The gown was too small, and I thought I'd break the sleeves as I bent over and put on my black socks, the green garment tight at the elbows and bunching up under my armpits. The bottom didn't even cover my knees, and I was glad to be wearing shorts, because the lower portion of my rear end was clearly out in the open. I left the exam room and went through the double doors again to x ray, my left hand grasping the front of the gown above my navel as I tapped the wall of the hallway every so often with my right. I felt ridiculous again. Here was a big football player, waiting for a flight to go play national powerhouse Michigan, dressed in black

socks, skivvy shorts, and a green hospital coat that was slit
open down the middle, too tight, and way too short. I passed
too many people in the hall and half ran, half skipped to
quickly close the door of the x-ray room behind me.

"You're the Navy football player, huh?" the technician on
duty asked as he was fiddling with the machine. I engaged
the corpsman in casual conversation all throughout various
positions on the table beneath the x-ray device, talking about
Navy's chances against Michigan, the top ten, and some of
the better college players. I mentioned the Penn State blowout
and John Cappelletti.

"Yeah, Cappelletti's tough, man. You think this Dorsett is
going to be anything? He's just a freshman—like you." The
corpsman was grinning as he took the last x ray.

"I don't know about Dorsett, but I do know I've got to get
out of here. I'm supposed to catch a flight this afternoon."

"Right on, man. You take care, now."

"See you later."

I took a look down the hall. Luckily there weren't too
many people this time, and I held the robe tightly in the center and walked briskly back to the urology examining room.

I stood in the windowless room, facing the door, the
green gown hanging on the dressing curtain, my t-shirt
placed on top of my shoes, skivvies again my only attire. I'd
been at Bethesda for more than two hours, and it was almost
3:00; I was growing impatient and had no idea where my
driver was. I remembered I didn't have my cover and needed
to talk to the driver to get both my hat and athletic bag. I was
annoyed, scared, and excited—this wasn't part of the usual
plebe routine, and playing against Michigan wasn't part of the
normal routine, either.

Dr. Leftwich finally came back, and I glanced at my watch
as he closed the door.

"I've taken a look at your x rays. We need to do a biopsy."

"A biopsy?"

"That's a routine surgical procedure, exploratory, where we go in and see what's in there."

I wondered what he was talking about. "You mean you're going to do an operation? Today?"

This was a direct challenge, and he was screwing up my plans. I had too much at stake and was not going to miss Michigan. Why did Eichelberger send me out here to Bethesda? Dr. Landry said everything could wait. What about Coach Welsh? This Dr. Leftwich didn't understand. How come I had to listen to him? We could do this Monday.

"Uh, doctor, you see, I . . . I play for Navy. I'm on the varsity. We're playing Michigan tomorrow, and I'm supposed to catch a flight later today and meet everybody there. They left a couple of hours ago, at 1:00. They've got my tickets and everything."

The doctor didn't say anything as I tried to explain the situation.

"There's a Navy driver waiting for me outside. Coach Welsh knows all about it. Couldn't we do this Monday, and take care of it then?"

I leaned out of the chair, Dr. Leftwich standing impassively by the closed door, and pleaded with him.

"I've got to go to the game, Dr. Leftwich. I'm going to start tomorrow. There're people waiting for me up there. The driver's waiting for me. I've got to get to the airport. Why can't we do this Monday? Nothing is going to happen. It can wait."

"No."

I sat back in my chair. What was happening?

"Tom, we need to see what's in there. A biopsy is a routine procedure. But it is imperative that we do it now. It is absolutely necessary."

I said nothing at first, looking at Leftwich, who just stood there with his arms folded.

"Whose decision is this?"

"Here at Bethesda, we operate, at least here in urology, with a staff review of a patient's preliminary diagnosis. The other doctors and I have reviewed your x rays, and based on that and my examination of you, and, of course, your medical record, we feel that an immediate biopsy is required."

"Today?"

"Today, Tom."

"Whose decision is this? Couldn't this wait till Monday?"

"It's my decision, along with our department. We make all decisions here as a group."

"I'd like to talk with the group, Doctor. I need to get another opinion. Why can't I wait until Monday? I feel fine."

"You need a biopsy today," Leftwich responded curtly, turning to leave. "It's a simple operation. Wait here. I'll see who's available to talk with you."

I remained seated. What was going on? How could I persuade these people to wait? I shifted uncomfortably in the chair, not embarrassed but angry and upset when the other staff finally arrived.

Six doctors in a semicircle faced me as I sat alone, naked, all personally examining me and all agreeing on the diagnosis and on a biopsy—today. I looked at each doctor closely; their faces matched the sterility of the room. What were they telling me? Why do they have to do it now? It's all a group opinion? I had an ominous feeling looking up at the serious faces of these older, professional men. Only a few hours before, it had been a completely different situation. I had been getting dressed for warmup drills and everything was so casual, so loose, a good day. Now—exploratory surgery? Things had still been on track even after Dr. Eichelberger had sent me to Bethesda. A commercial ticket was neat, something different, and Susie McElroy would have definitely been impressed. Now—an operation? Was something wrong? I wasn't thinking anymore of my aching testicle. I had to go to Michigan. It was a chance for plenty of game time. How could I convince them they could wait until Monday? Biopsy? Exploratory surgery? What were they talking about? I wanted to get up and leave.

All of the doctors concurred. "You should have a biopsy." Each one. They'd introduced themselves when Leftwich brought them in, but I'd forgotten their names. I didn't care about their credentials—did they really know what it was they were interfering with? But they didn't seem to care— they just stood there, cool and detached.

I sat straight up in the chair and looked furtively at the physicians who stood around me. Who was I to tell them no? A plebe? I felt like disappointment had been injected directly into my heart.

"I think we should call my dad first. I mean, before you operate . . . before the, uh, biopsy."

"I'll take care of that," Leftwich responded.

The group left the room. Dr. Leftwich was the last to leave, looking back before he closed the door. I thought he was going to say something, but he looked away and the door shut. I sat alone on the chair. The room was cold.

CHAPTER THREE

The chartered aircraft carrying the Navy football team was being pushed back from the ramp when the Naval Academy superintendent, Vice Admiral William P. Mack, felt a tap on his shoulder. Adjusting his seatbelt and turning sideways, Admiral Mack looked at Bo Coppidge, the athletic director, who was shaking his head slowly.

"What's the matter, Bo?"

"Well, Admiral, Tommy Harper probably has cancer."

Admiral Mack had been a tight end for Coach Tom Harlin years before at Navy, and he took a personal interest in the football team, the coaches giving him a list of the players during the summer drills, what positions they could play, and who were the best athletes. He was quiet as the ground gave way, the runway lost to sight when the pilot banked the plane toward the northwest with a gently rolling motion. What Coppidge had to say cast a pall over the start of the trip. They were at cruise altitude over the checkerboard terrain below when he looked back at the athletic director and said, "Tom's got a chance."

I dressed slowly, putting my service dress-blue uniform back on as meticulously as I had done before. It was hard to accept their decision, but I thought that if I was lucky I might get out on a later flight or maybe on one early the next morning. Game time wasn't until the early afternoon, so there was still plenty of time to get there. I buttoned the last gold clasp on my blouse, adjusted my cuffs, and opened the door.

The driver was waiting by the receptionist's desk and handed me my overnight bag and white, black-billed hat.

"How are you doing? You left these in the car."

"Thanks. I've got to go to admissions now. They want to do a biopsy today. I hope it's quick."

The receptionist repeated the directions to admissions, and the driver and I walked there together. How could I get out of this? Michigan was on my mind as I filled out "Harper, Thomas J." on the hospital forms. I hesitantly resigned myself to disappointment, but maybe there was a chance, still time to get to Michigan.

I was directed to the eleventh floor in the main shaft, tower 11, and we rode the elevator up in silence until the floor was highlighted by an amber light above the doors. "This must be it," I said, the corpsman shrugging in agreement. With one step out of the elevator, we could see the nursing station.

"I'm Midshipman Harper."

"Thomas Harper?"

"Yes, Ma'am."

"Yes, we've got you in 1119. Please follow me."

My driver wished me good luck and then took the elevator back down to the first floor and headed for the parking lot.

"You'll have to get undressed."

I turned around, the voice of another corpsman surprising me.

"We have to do a tit-to-thigh on you."

"What's that?"

"We have to shave you from here," the corpsman said, pointing to the top of his chest, "to here," bending over to touch his knee.

"Yeah, but you're only operating here," I retorted, pointing to my groin.

"Please, it's required. It's done all the time," he replied, continuing with an explanation that angered me as I opened a closet door and undressed.

I lay naked on the single bed along the far wall of room 1119, the corpsman's hand unnatural and cold on my chest. I felt vulnerable and awkward as I watched his every move. The shaving was painless, but I felt violated again, the corpsman's hands out of place on my body as he expertly moved the razor in the glare of the light overhead. Why didn't they just let me do this myself? I knew right then that there was no way I was going to Michigan—these people were serious.

The shower water was refreshing at first, but the betadine soap solution took all the pleasure out of it, pellets of water running down my back to mix with the brownish-red fluid that dripped from my hands. The betadine, oily and odorless, had no lather, and I had to rinse off twice to get rid of the slimy coat it left on my skin. It was strange not to have any pubic hair.

"Tom, I'm Dr. Prough, your anesthetist."

I turned from looking out the single, small window in my room.

"Let's go over a few things, OK?"

Dr. Prough had a casual, relaxed manner, and there was a pleasant inflection to his voice that made me like him immediately.

"I bet you never thought you'd be here today, huh?"

"No, that's for sure."

"Have a seat. I've got a few things I want to go over with you regarding the anesthetic procedure. It's fairly straightforward. We can give you a local or put you out completely." He went on to finish explaining how a local would be administered through a spinal injection of pontocaine.

"What's pontocaine?"

"It's a drug similar to novocaine. You know, the dentist . . ." Dr. Prough opened his mouth in a wide grin and pointed a finger toward his gums.

"A shot in the back, huh?"

"Your lower back, Tom," he replied, turning around and running his fingers along the small curve of his backside. "It deadens everything from here on down. The lumbar area here."

"Yes, let's go with that. I'd like to see what's going on."

"Good show. I'll see you in a bit. You'll do fine."

Dr. Prough grinned, patted me on the shoulder, and left.

I felt comfortable with him and adjusted the blue pinstriped
robe they'd given me to wear as I rested on the edge of my
bed.

"Are you Midshipman Harper?"
"Yes."
"You've got a telephone call in the doctor's office."
I followed the nurse down the hall to a small office where
a doctor had put the call on hold.
"I'm Dr. Timmons. I believe your father is on the line."
"Thank you," I replied, nodding in appreciation as Dr.
Timmons left and softly shut the door.
My father is an incredibly strong man emotionally, and all
throughout my childhood he was always there to say the right
words or provide a firm hand to grasp. I love and respect him
and usually tried to do what he would expect me to do, no
matter what the circumstance. Dad was a quiet, comforting
man while I was growing up, and the sense of his presence
remains with me to this day.
"Dad?"
"You've got a little problem out there, son? How are you
doing?"
"Listen, Dad, don't worry. They say it's a routine operation, and I should be out pretty soon. Ah, I don't think we
should tell Mom anything until we find out exactly . . . you
know . . . OK?"
"All right, Tommy."
"Did Dr. Leftwich call you?"
"Yes, just a few minutes ago."
"That's good. That's good." I wanted to tell him every-
thing I thought, but I was groping for something to say.
"How's everything in San Mateo?"
"Just fine. Your mother's at work now."
"I'd better get going, Dad. I'll call you as soon as every-
thing is over."
"Just relax, Tommy. You'll do fine."
"OK. See you."
I put down the receiver slowly, opened the door, and
went back to room 1119. I felt better after talking with my

father. His calm, reassuring voice always made hard things seem to go a little easier. It felt funny to rub my hand over my chest and abdomen, the absence of body hair giving me a diaphanous feeling, but at least my new robe wasn't as embarrassing as the green one I'd first worn to x ray.

It was only a matter of minutes until a dolly was rolled into the room by another corpsman.

"You can leave your bathrobe here. We're going to wrap you in these sheets."

I slipped out of the robe, placing it on the bed, and stood naked again, feeling clumsy. Dr. Prough's presence at the door only slightly relieved my anxiety.

I trembled as the needle was inserted into my spine, and grasped the rails of my dolly as it was withdrawn. I didn't like needles and shots, and I didn't like standing naked in front of people for the third time today. When the stainless steel guards were locked into place, it seemed a signal that whatever was happening was now out of my control. Jesus, I thought, I hope they cover me up; surely they wouldn't push me naked through the hall and down the elevator.

"We're headed to the operating room now, Tom." It was Dr. Prough, who adjusted the corner of one sheet over my leg as the corpsman finished wrapping me, the sheets fresh and clean.

The elevator doors opened to the second floor, and I thought that everybody in the hospital was looking at me. Jesus Christ, what are these people thinking? Dr. Prough gently slapped my face to keep me alert and stopped the dolly just outside the operating room door to administer an IV, a sharp twinge going through my body as we went through the doorway.

"I laughed at a guy who once had this done to him," I said to Prough.

"That's normal, Tom."

It was hard to stay awake, and Dr. Prough gently tapped my face as a white curtain was drawn up in front of me. I was supposed to watch the operation and mumbled, "Hey, wait a minute," but they put another curtain in front of my eyes, and I felt dizzy and sick and remember being slapped lightly in the face before blacking out completely. Maybe they tried to keep me awake.

My chart described a fully developed, 19-year-old, white male with a testicular mass. Testicular tumors are usually a young man's disease, and Dr. Leftwich held out hope that the diagnosis would be benign, as the possible result of malignancy weighed heavily on him.

He'd received an earlier call from Dr. Clancy at the Academy, and unless it was absolutely vital, Clancy saw no reason to keep me at the hospital over the weekend. This Michigan game could be the only game I'd have a chance to play.

"Please let this kid play one damned game. You're only talking about two damned days," Dr. Clancy had said to him. Leftwich explained that an immediate operation could make a difference; therapy could get started sooner.

"Well, you're a urologist, and I'm an orthopedist. I'm not going to argue with you . . . yet . . . well, if you feel it's vital . . ."

"We must operate today," Leftwich repeated again, and after a momentary silence, Clancy agreed it was the right thing to do.

Jesus Christ, it's all over for the kid, Clancy thought. He knew the prognosis for testicular cancer was especially poor. Malignancy was not new to him, and Dr. Clancy remembered his cousin's treatment for a similar disease. The chemotherapy took all his cousin's vigor, his hair—he was emaciated. It was difficult to watch anyone being poisoned, and his cousin had died.

It was a 50-minute operation. Dr. Leftwich placed his scalpel on my lower left abdomen, paralleling the ligament and pushing deep down to connective tissue. The spermatic cord was isolated and clamped, and my left testes was delivered into the wound, examined, dissected, freed from my scrotum, and removed. The operational procedure went well; vital signs were normal; the anesthetist indicated to Dr. Leftwich that I was fast asleep. There was about 100 ccs of clear fluid surrounding the testicle, which was swollen and full, triple the normal size. Dr. Leftwich would wait until the pathology report to talk to me, but he already knew what he would have to say. Leftwich telephoned my dad within the hour after I was wheeled into recovery.

"I've just operated on Tom and pulled out a tumor of pretty good size. Although we've not yet performed the lab tests, I can tell you right now it's malignant. I don't think his prognosis will be favorable."

"How's he doing?"

"He's in satisfactory condition. He's in recovery and will remain there overnight."

"When will the biopsy report be ready, Doctor?"

"We should have the pathologist's report by Monday. I'll call you when I receive word."

"Please, Doctor . . . goodbye."

Dad was dumbfounded. This never happens to us; this doesn't happen to Tommy, he thought to himself—besides, they'd just seen me during Parents' Weekend. It just doesn't happen at all. He wondered what could be done, but there was nothing he could do, medically anyway, and there was certainly nothing I could do at the moment. He thanked God that I was in a place where people cared for people, and said a silent prayer.

The telephone was ringing as my 14-year-old brother Richard came walking through the front door of our house in San Mateo. He'd just completed Friday's football practice, and for a brief moment he was tempted to forget about the telephone and instead fix himself a nice, big sandwich. But the phone wouldn't stop ringing, so he reluctantly picked up the receiver.

"Hello."

"Is this the Harper residence?"

"Yes, it is."

"Is Mr. or Mrs. Harper there?"

"No. They'll be home in about an hour. Can I take a message?"

"Well, yes. This is George Welsh, Tommy's football coach."

"Oh, yeah?" Richard's interest picked up immediately. He played linebacker, all five foot eight, 140 pounds of him, and it wasn't that often he talked with a college football coach.

"Tom's at the Bethesda Naval Hospital. He couldn't make the Michigan trip. I understand they've operated on him for a groin tumor. It's not been determined if it's malignant or benign. Maybe the doctors have talked with your folks already. I'm not sure." Coach Welsh concluded the conversation with a brief description of what had happened before my admission, saying that I was resting well at Bethesda. George said he'd be back in touch, and Richard thanked him for calling as he hung up the phone. I'd called home a couple of days before to tell everybody I'd get my chance Saturday, and Rich was disappointed that I wouldn't be playing now.

The long Plymouth wagon pulled up out front at its regular hour, the engine coughing, sputtering, and finally dying as the ponderous machine leaned against the curb. Richard was halfway to the front door when it opened, my 17-year-old sister Theresa, a senior at my old alma mater Oceana High School, and my mother coming into the house.

"George Welsh called and said Tommy's in the hospital with a tumor or something. He said he'd call back." He was surprised by their reaction. Tommy'd been sick before. What's the big deal? Mom had suddenly changed, her habitually relaxed, cheerful expression becoming serious and concerned. It hurts, still, to think of her having to hear such news. She, like my father, is a special person, a woman whose perseverance and compassion has left a soft and beautiful place in my soul.

Theresa was quiet at first, which was unusual, given her gregarious and friendly personality.

"A tumor? What did he say, Richard? What kind of tumor? Is it malignant? Where is it?"

"I don't know, Theresa. Big deal. He said he'd call back."

Mom interrupted, "All right, all right. Now, Rich, what exactly did Coach Welsh say?" My brother repeated the conversation as clearly as he could remember it but still wondered what they were so concerned about. Mom was quiet as she went about the house, but Rich could tell she was worried, and Theresa made him look up *tumor* and *malignant* in the dictionary.

Dad arrived home early, and my parents talked quietly together, nobody saying much around the table, and everyone ate slowly. The long table seemed extra empty, and something was bugging Mom and Dad, but Rich didn't want to intrude.

Coach Welsh called my parents later that same evening, and Rich, alone in his room reading *Sports Illustrated*, could hear the tail end of their conversation. It wasn't a long call.

"Should we call Mary Beth?"

"No, dear, I don't think so. She's supposed to call tomorrow, you know. We can talk about it then."

"Are you going out to the boat in the morning?"

"I'm not sure. Let's see what develops."

Rich put his magazine down, left his room, and knocked softly on their door.

"Mom?"

"Yes, Richard."

"Is Tommy going to be all right?"

"He's in good hands, son. Just think of him in your prayers."

Theresa was still awake, reading in the living room.

"It's really serious, huh?" he said to her.

"It could be, Richard. If the tumor is malignant, that means he has cancer."

"That's pretty bad, huh? Tommy can't have cancer. He's in too good of shape for that."

"Cancer doesn't care what kind of shape you're in, Richard," Theresa replied softly, and they sat in silence for a few minutes. Rich turned on the small black and white television, where a smiling news announcer was talking with a fat weatherman. Bored, he pulled the plug and went to sleep.

The Michigan hotel lobby wasn't crowded, and not many people were at the registration desk, just a few feet from where Sandra Welsh was sitting. It was quiet the night before the game, and Sandra shared her husband's intensity for the next day's contest.

Red Romo was talking to Dr. Eichelberger. Sandra smiled upon seeing their friendly faces across the lobby. She saw Red acknowledge something to the team doctor, but Marty had his back to her, and he entered an elevator as she got up and walked across the lobby. Red gave a chagrined look when he saw her approach, the elevator door closing behind them. He had told her earlier that I'd missed the flight, saying only that I had to go to Bethesda to get a groin injury checked.

"One of our ball players has cancer."

"Tommy Harper?"

"Yes, they've removed a tumor. Marty says they think it's malignant."

"Dear God."

"George has talked to his parents. I think he's calling some of Tommy's friends now who were supposed to meet him here."

In nearby Tecumseh, Ken McElroy could hear his 18-year-old daughter crying alone in her room, and he hesitated to open her door. She'd been on the phone, and perhaps this was a private matter, but something told him to intrude.

"What's wrong, Susie?" She was lying on her bed, tears running down her pretty face, sobbing quietly as her father took her in his arms and hugged her while she told him what George Welsh had to say. He wanted to meet them after the game.

I stayed in recovery overnight. The hospital had treated several testicular cancer patients, and Nurse Chris Picchi had cared for many of them in her two years at Bethesda. My operation results were like many of the others—a three- to six-month prognosis at best.

The small transistor radio next to my ear made a small hum. I felt groggy, and it was dark, but I could make out my anesthetist, Dr. Prough, a nurse, and a corpsman standing around me. The lower half of my body was numb. I moved my left leg but couldn't seem to put it back down. Awake, I realized I hadn't been able to move the leg at all.

"Did you take it out?"

"Yes." Was that Prough that responded? Who were these people standing around my bed? What time was it? Were nurses with me now?

"Did Navy win?" I started to get up, but a gentle hand slowly lowered me back to the pillow.

"Stay still. You don't need a headache later on. Just gentle movements."

The feminine voice was sweet, refreshing, and calm, and as the nurse adjusted the sound of the radio, I closed my eyes and relaxed.

I could feel the bandage over my groin and lower abdomen and knew I was going to feel better. I'd asked one of the doctors before the operation how long I'd be in the hospital. Dr. Timmons replied that I'd be ready to go in six days—three days till I was up and three more till I could run. I'd be walking around by Monday, and after a couple of light practices would be at full speed by Thursday; we were playing Syracuse that Saturday, and I would be ready for that. I was disappointed about missing the Michigan game but happy at least that the nagging hurt would soon be gone. I felt weak, obviously from the operation, and my groin was tender. I was looking forward to calling home and telling everybody I was OK.

Luckily, I hadn't missed any classes. I knew plebe year, even with all its headaches, wouldn't last forever. It was certainly better than having to stay at Bethesda, and I was determined to get back on course. I wanted to find out the score of the Michigan game, but mostly I was glad everything was finally over. All was well.

CHAPTER FOUR

There was pressure building in the back of my head, and I adjusted my neck on the pillow, the discomfort leaving briefly but then growing in intensity. The clock on the wall across from my mobile bed read 10:58 P.M. I felt sick and closed my eyes, the ache more intense, becoming a steady throb in my brain. I tried to concentrate on the music coming from the small radio, but the sounds were intermittent. Looking straight up, I could see the exposed ceiling pipes that ran at right angles to my legs. Three or four hours must have elapsed before I heard a man talking, the wall clock visible over his right shoulder. It read 11:02 P.M.—only four minutes had gone by.

"Can you feel your legs? Your knees?"

"I'm not sure. Are you sticking me with a pin?"

"Try to raise your legs."

I couldn't. I tried three times, sure that they were up, but nothing moved. The corpsman kept squeezing my knees, and I felt a burning sensation in my thighs. Was he sticking me with a pin, or what? I adjusted myself sideways in the bed, my abdomen and groin stiff under the bandage, my calves tight as I tried to stretch out my legs. The anesthetic was wearing off, I was getting some movement back, and, thankfully, I noticed my headache was starting to ebb.

"I can feel some of my legs now," I said to the corpsman. "How long will it take for all of this to wear off?"

"Shouldn't take too long. You'll be fine by morning." He smiled and went about his other business, leaving me alone.

Friday had been a long day for Chris Picchi, and she was looking forward to calling it a night. My chart was on the small desk at her station, the words "football player" written next to my name, and it was sad to think that I was dying. She'd asked me something about Navy when I was conscious, but I'd just mumbled and gone back to sleep.

No one on her shift had eaten since breakfast, and Chris asked out loud, "Does anyone want to get something to eat?" The group of nurses discussed a couple of places outside the hospital where they could get pizza and beer.

"Can I come, too?" I said, still half asleep and raising myself so I could get out of bed.

"Can I come? I'm ready." Picchi came over, patted me softly on the forehead, and eased me back down to the mattress. I could feel her left hand behind my shoulder and her right hand on my arm. There was a gentleness to her touch.

"Hey, let me go. I'm hungry. I'm feeling better. I need to get up and walk around. I've missed too much already. I'll be out of here in a couple of days anyway. C'mon."

She stopped talking about food, and I just nodded and fell back to sleep. Picchi knew I didn't know what was going on, that I had cancer, that the surgery was serious—I wasn't as insistent flat on my back.

The Navy midshipmen were decided underdogs against the powerful Michigan Wolverines, but we were kept in the game by tough defensive play, losing only 14 to 7. Ken McElroy took Susie to the Navy locker room to talk with Coach Welsh, knowing it would be quite subdued after the loss, but Navy played much better than he had expected. George smiled as he introduced himself and touched Susie's shoulder mildly.

"Mr. McElroy? Hello, Susie, I'm George Welsh. I was asked to talk with you. That's why I called last night. I can only apologize if it caused you displeasure."

"We understand."

"It's too early to come to any conclusions. I understand there are more tests to run. They did remove a tumor. Tommy will be in the hospital for some time. Sandra?" George continued, looking at his wife, who had joined them.

"Hello, I'm Sandra Welsh," the attractive woman said as she gathered Susie to her in comfort.

"Here is our telephone number. Please call us. Our door is always open. We'll do everything we can to help."

I passed the night under careful observation, awakening in midmorning with the bandage still intact. I could flex my legs and lift them, but they were sore, and I still had a slight headache when they moved me back to the eleventh floor, tower 11, room 1119. I'd missed Michigan, but I'd done all I could do. It was still uncomfortable to think about that cold exam room, where the doctors had told me I could miss the whole season if my swollen testicle took a hard hit. I'd be out of here in a few days, and that thought eased me back to sleep.

My room was no bigger than the rooms in Bancroft, and it was accented by a harsh light that came out from between the sprinkler pipes installed on the ceiling. The wall behind me was painted green, the rest of the walls were a dirty beige color, and there was a window by the bathroom door that needed cleaning. I felt very tired, not caring if I ever got up. The picture tube of the TV was blank and gray, and every now and then I'd recognize my roommate, but I couldn't see him too well. It felt better just to keep my eyes closed.

The bathroom was shared with the adjoining room, and the door would frequently open and close. Someone would use the toilet, and I could hear every drop of water in the pipes, accented by a glimpse of a thin bead of light escaping from the bottom of the door. Doctors, corpsmen, and nurses would come in and out, and I could feel their hands lifting the covers, taking my pulse, touching my forehead. I remembered Dr. Timmons and a Dr. Grady coming in—both were friendly and smiled, but I couldn't recall what they had to say.

My parents waited for the pathology report. Dad called the hospital, and they told him I would be in bed all weekend and that, so far, I was sleeping peacefully. Mom explained to all seven of my brothers and sisters scattered across the country what had happened, trading concern quietly as everybody waited for more definitive news. It wasn't easy for her to tell everyone what had happened. She drew some comfort in their reaction, though, as the whole family surrounded her with understanding and quiet support.

My parents left for the boatyard, a 45-minute drive that had become a weekend ritual. "Latare," they called it, Latin for "joy," a 50-foot, two-masted ketch, a sailor's dream. My father had carefully built it by himself, with his own sure hands. Everyone in our family had gotten the word, but Mom still couldn't tell them everything, and they all helped by not asking too much. She wondered if I knew yet what was really wrong. She patted Dad's hand, and he smiled slightly, glancing toward the still water of the bay under the San Mateo bridge. It was a terrible heartache to be so far away.

Saturday had come and was almost gone. The early afternoon sun bathed the other end of the room, dust particles dancing in the cubed shafts of light by the bathroom door. My mouth was dry, but the cold juice, placed on the vanity next to me while I was asleep, relieved some of the fatigue as I swished it around inside my mouth.

I was surprised to see Phil Nelson come in. I had met him in late October of 1972 while we were both at NAPS, and he had become a close friend. Football season was almost over then, and I was debating whether to play basketball or to start serious weight training in preparation for my first real season of college football, coming up in less than a year. Phil, fresh out of high school like myself, was a good basketball player and already a standout in preseason. He'd been studying, seated at his desk, the low beating sound of a desk clock accompanying the mundane material in front of him. I'd opened his door and looked in at him, my leering face interrupting his concentration. There were just a few of us in the company who played football. Here's another cocky "sonofabitch," Phil thought, staring at me.

"Do you mind if I ask you a question?" I said. I'd never spoken to him before.

"No."

"Do you think I should go out for basketball?"

Phil knew who I was, and I'd heard he was a pretty good

basketball player, but he'd never said a word to me either, until just now. Grace us with your presence, he thought, as he looked at me with bored resignation, then turned his head back to continue reading. Not looking up, he replied, "I don't give a damn what you do."

"Oh."

I closed the door, puzzled that he hadn't bothered to look up again, and wondered, who is this guy? It was surprising that we worked as well as we did together in practice later on, perhaps because we weren't competing for the same position. We had plenty of one-on-one games and a running rivalry with our scoring averages. The NAPS team won as many games as it lost, and we both started for a team that was good one day and mediocre the next. We developed a close friendship, and the season was fun regardless of the final score. Phil and I played good basketball and shared numerous exploits around the Prep School campus.

"Hey, Tom. How are you doing?" Phil asked as he patted me on the leg. Gordy McElroy, Susie's brother and another close friend, was right behind him.

"How'd you guys get here?"

"We got a chit and drove out. No problem. You doing OK?"

"I guess so. I'm tired, but I should be . . . out of here in a couple of days." I tried to sit up, but it felt much better to stay down, and although Phil was surprised by my weak handshake, he didn't show any worry. We talked about Plebe Summer, not having seen much of each other since the day before the swearing-in ceremony. Nobody mentioned anything about cancer. Some of the upperclass football players came by shortly after Phil and Gordy; our starting quarterback Al Glenny, the team captain Charlie Miletich, and our All-American safety Chet Moeller, telling me all about the game.

"Fourteen to seven? Must have been a great game. I'd like to see the films," I said, and Chet replied he'd bring it up with the coaches.

It was good to talk with everybody. I'd close my eyes, and it seemed like there were many more people in my room. I tried to thank everybody and drifted off for a moment, the sunlight gone when I awoke, a hall light illuminating the backside of the room door. My roommate wasn't there, a couple of chairs were pulled up around my bed, and I vaguely recalled talking to some mids. Had Phil been here? It was dark outside, and there was no sound to the night as I went back to sleep.

Dr. Leftwich reviewed my case history early Monday morning, the medical file indicating Naval Academy physicians had treated me for epididymis (sperm blockage) with limited success.

The surgery Friday evening was normal, and I'd tolerated the procedure well, losing only 75 ccs of blood. The tumor was malignant—he was sure of it, and my protocol would be based on the definitive findings of the pathology report. In the interim, there were tests to schedule to help in determining how far the disease had spread, because metastasis was potentially fatal and could lead to progressive failure of body organs and other unpleasant complications. He wrote the list in the medical record:

Blood culture	2 ea
Chest x rays	2 ea
Liver scan	2 ea
Bone scan	2 ea
Gallium scan	2 ea
Inferior vena cava gram	2 ea
Lymphangiogram	2 ea
Chest tomogram	2 ea

Leftwich reflected over his previous notes, noting "Emergency Orchiectomy," which he'd written that Friday afternoon. It would still be a couple of days until definite word from pathology, and he'd often use this time to allow things to settle with his patients, who were usually stunned by the operation. My initial convalescence appeared to have been peaceful, and I was resting quietly when he visited tower 11 over the weekend.

Monday breakfast came early, but I was awake, the weekend over, thinking that I'd be getting ready for class about now and wondering what *The Washington Post* had to say about the game.

"Tom?"

I recognized the soft-spoken voice of Dr. Leftwich, who was at the doorway to the room, leaning against the frame but standing almost in the hall.

"These next few days are going to be very tiring for you. We'll need your understanding and patience. You'll be up early in the morning all week . . . long days, very tiring, you know . . . test after test after test. You'll be tired, but you've got to keep going." He shrugged and left.

I'd raised myself up in the bed to hear the doctor better, but he hadn't come into the room. What were the tests for? The operation was over; the anesthetic had worn off; I didn't have a headache and had slept well overnight. Anyway, I was ready to leave, and I wanted to tell him so. My groin was tender, the bandages were two days old, and I felt weak, but this had to pass. I was getting better and would be back with the brigade this week. I had to get out of bed and walk around. Leftwich obviously didn't know what was going on.

"Get up, get up. You've got to get up. C'mon. You've got to get started." My mattress was shaking. It was still dark outside, the light on the ceiling, however, focusing directly into my eyes. The nurse looked remarkably awake, her uniform white and freshly pressed. I remember looking at her but never recall her ever entering the room. She'd appear out of nowhere every day, just to wake me up.

The cold water was invigorating as it washed the stale skin from my face. I couldn't completely shower because the wound was too recent, but with my breath refreshed and teeth clean, I looked at myself in the mirror. I looked the same as I did before the operation, and I still had the other testicle.

There were nurses going here and there in tower 11, and I'd see a doctor or two. I didn't feel like a plebe back at Bancroft Hall, and it was nice to talk with relative freedom to people walking around the ward. Life was back in my legs, and I could stretch a little and even bend over to touch the tips of my toes. I looked forward to working out again, impatient to get whatever tests Dr. Leftwich was talking about over with, and quickly, because I couldn't waste any more time getting ready for the Syracuse game on Saturday. More importantly, perhaps, I had to catch up in class.

I skipped breakfast, and a corpsman pushed me in a wheelchair down from tower 11 to begin all the tests. I was taken back by the double doors leading to one test room: "Hazard Area—Nuclear Radiation," the sign said, the yellow and black print stripes contrasting with the mute color of the corridor. I flinched at the insertion of needles and stood, often, in front of heavy cold machines. The first few minutes went by fast, but it was always another hour before I could back off from the devices. The injections made me sick to my stomach. Some of the corpsmen tried to explain to me what they were doing.

"The injection was a radioisotope, and the machine traces it to your liver and spleen. We're checking for any complications."

"Oh." They'd have to push me back to my room.

I went into one darkened room and lay flat on a hard table, my blue pajama legs rolled up over my knees, a TV screen attached to the wall on my left, projecting light that gave a delicate glow to the stainless steel. There were two doctors by my feet, one on each side of the table, and I could see myself in the reflection of the younger man's wire-rimmed eyeglasses.

"We're going to make an incision just in front of your big toes, Tom. We'll identify a lymphatic vessel and slowly inject a dye. It should light up some lymph nodes, and we can trace them on the screen there." The older doctor nodded toward the television screen as he finished talking, and both physicians gave me local injections, the puncture pin sharp and piercing as my feet went numb. They were cutting three-inch slits in my feet.

The younger doctor was having some trouble, and I raised up on my elbows, grimacing at the sight of him pulling my skin apart, widening the wound as he looked for the right place to put his needle. The older doctor, giving instructions, saw me react and gave me another shot of novocaine in the right foot.

"I'm OK," I said as the point of another needle went through my skin.

"I'm OK," I repeated, lying back down on the table to follow the progress of the blue dye on the monitor screen.

"I don't feel anything."

The bone scan machine gave out a steady hum as it moved back and forth, covering every inch of me and brushing my chest every other pass. I couldn't move under that machine, and the only thing I could see in the room was a cabinet full of blood vials. My muscles ached like they did after a hard workout on the practice field or from lifting weights.

I'd wait for an hour, receive another radioisotope injection, wait another hour, and then find myself on a long table, another strange machine scanning my abdomen, the technician saying they were looking for enlarged lymph nodes. There were more liver and spleen scans, more bone scans, gallium scans, lymphangiograms, brain scans. I was wheeled back and forth to x ray, where they kept telling me they were taking pictures of my lungs in different areas and levels. Once that was completed, they took blood samples. Every day they were taking samples.

I got back to my room late. My feet were blue and sore, and I walked carefully, not able to keep weight on them too long, and a corpsman helped me back into bed. Dr. Leftwich had been in and out since Monday, and I was getting different kinds of medication at different times of the day, my diet was off, and it was hard to keep an appetite. It was hell getting to sleep, and I felt sick most of the time. I hadn't shaved in six days, and I was tired, drawnout, and wondered what was next. I hadn't eaten much at all since the weekend, and it had been five days since I'd worked out and even longer since I'd studied. I was falling way behind in academics, the books in my overnight bag still unopened in the closet. I would have to catch up and explain all of this to my profs. My company officer had been by earlier to visit and found me in tower IV, sitting in my wheelchair by a water fountain, waiting, as usual, for more tests. I'd have to practice hard to be in condition for the remainder of the season, and an hour didn't go by when I wasn't thinking about the team going through scrimmages. I was tired of the x rays, tired of sitting around waiting in wheelchairs, tired of "Breathe deep. Hold it. Relax." I'd lost count of how long and how many times I'd been in front of machines. I knew I was losing weight. My arms felt flabby, I had no energy, I was always sleepy—what the hell was happening to me?

One morning while waiting to be wheeled to yet another test, a wheelchair came rolling slowly toward me from the other end of the hall. I was surprised to see it held a little boy, not more than six years old, a skinny, pasty-white kid with a tiny neck, his bald head accentuating ears that looked too big.

"How're you doing?" I asked, forgetting for a moment my own problems.

"Just fine. Want to race?"

"Sure." The corpsman with me stepped aside, and the boy and I lined up abreast. Two turns of the wheels, and I'd have him beat, but I let him take the lead to the end of the corridor. He squealed happily all the way.

"All right!" I exclaimed. "You're pretty fast!"

"I've been doing this a lot, you know," he answered, scarcely above a whisper but with excitement in his eyes.

There were two crutches attached to the back of the boy's wheelchair, and I said, "I'll get a crutch tomorrow, and we'll sword fight." He nodded in agreement as the nurse on station came to get him.

"Bye-bye," the little boy said. He seemed strangely out of place in that wheelchair, as the nurse spun him around and down the hall.

I waited for him the next day, sitting in a wheelchair by the elevator with a crutch I'd found in a vacant room. The little boy was usually in the hall early in the afternoon.

"En garde!" The kid had his crutch out like a lance and was bearing down on me with a full head of steam. I wheeled out into the corridor and caught the rubber tip square in the chest, the boy dropping it on impact.

"Ugggh!" I shouted. "You got me!" I put my hands over my heart and dropped my head down. He trembled as we traded blows back and forth, and I had to continually pick up his crutch because he couldn't hold it up too long.

The nurse with the youngster watched from down the hall. Here was a midshipman, oversized for the wheelchair, trading laughs with a boy who didn't weigh more than 40 pounds. If she listened hard, she could hear that distinctive little laughter the cancer would never take away.

"Midshipman Harper, it's time for another test," she said, her words stopping the duel. The boy was exhausted. I went to my room to wash up, feeling rejuvenated after playing around with my little friend. I returned to the nurses' station later to pick up my chart, and another corpsman took me to the elevator. When it opened on the bottom floor, I saw the little boy with his nurse getting into the elevator right next to us.

"Hey!" I shouted.

The boy moved only his eyes at first, but then his fingers moved and he struggled to wave, managing a lingering smile as the elevator doors opened and the nurse pushed him inside. She was kind enough to hold the doors open, and the corpsman and I waited until he gave us a tiny wave. I could only smile back at him, and the elevator doors closed when he slumped over in his wheelchair. I never saw that little boy again.

Dr. Leftwich knew the disease had spread. The test results were mostly positive—the liver and spleen scan, the lymphangiogram, initial chest x rays—they were not favorable. Drug treatment was required immediately.

Leftwich read the biopsy report twice, the pathologist confirming his earlier diagnosis, the last two lines of the report set apart from the preceding text:

> Excision left testes and spermatic cord: seminoma with embryonal carcinoma.

Leftwich recognized both from the test results and the confirmed biopsy that I would be fortunate to celebrate my twentieth birthday, less than 45 days away.

He closed my file and picked up the syringe from the small tray in front of him, slowly rotating the pointed instrument with both hands. This would be my first chemotherapy treatment, and I'd become a different person the moment the needle was pushed into my skin. The yellowish-gold antinomycin is foreign to the body, a toxic drug that affects patients in different ways but with a commonality of nausea and unpleasantness. I was big, strong, and in excellent physical condition when I checked into the hospital, and it was dissatisfying to Dr. Leftwich to have to change that.

The doctor put the syringe back down and depressed a metal tab in his address file to find my father's business number. It was 10:00 A.M. in the Bay area.

Dad was alone in his office and responded to the first ring of the telephone. "Jack Harper."

"Mr. Harper? This is Frederick Leftwich, Dr. Leftwich from Bethesda."

"Oh, yes, Doctor, have you found out anything?" Dad asked, sitting forward on the edge of his chair, straining to pick up every word.

"Yes, Mr. Harper, we have. It's, ah, rather unpleasant news, but . . . does confirm what I told you earlier about the malignancy. The biopsy report was . . . positive . . . and this merely confirms our initial opinion. It . . ."

"How's Tom today?" Dad interrupted.

"Well, he's been resting comfortably and undergoing the series of tests we talked about Monday. He's in good spirits."

"So, the biopsy report did confirm the tumor is malignant? Correct, Doctor?"

"Yes, Mr. Harper, that it did."

"What's the next step . . . ah . . ." My father could not continue, and there was an awkward silence while he relaxed his grip on the telephone handle, his knuckles white but then returning to their normal color.

"We'll begin initial chemotherapy today, Jack. Tom will be under an initial five-day program. He'll be taking several

more tests. We're going to concentrate with lung involvement. His liver and spleen scan were positive, and the
lymphangiogram did show some blockage. So there has been
some spread of cancer." Dr. Leftwich patiently repeated the
interpretation of all the various tests, concluding that he'd be
getting back in touch by the weekend.

The line went dead, and my father hung up. This still
doesn't happen to us, he thought again. He had pleasant
thoughts and memories of all his children, and cancer was
difficult to accept. There was only so much a man could do,
and he gave his thoughts to God.

Dr. Leftwich was supposed to see me Thursday afternoon, and I anticipated he'd tell me the tests were over and
that I'd be getting out of the hospital. I was in my room at 2:00
P.M., lying in bed when he came to the door but not saying
anything in greeting. I'd been talking to my new roommate, a
gentleman in his sixties from nearby Chevy Chase, Maryland,
who left the room to leave me alone with Leftwich.

I adjusted my pajamas. I wore a different pair each day,
and sometimes the pants were too short or the waist too big,
and one day I'd have buttons, the next day none, but the material was always fresh and unsoiled. Dr. Leftwich was carrying a syringe and a rubber tourniquet on a small tray, the
syringe full of a sickly looking fluid. I didn't say anything as
he approached me.

"Let me see your arm, Tom. What I'm going to do is to
give you this injection. It's called chemotherapy."

"Another shot," I said out loud, tired of the medication.

There was hard compression to the tourniquet as he tied
the rubber strip tightly behind my upper bicep, the veins in
my arm visible and popping up as I made a fist. Dr. Leftwich
checked the syringe and dabbed at my arm with a small cot-
ton ball, the alcohol moist to my skin, a shimmer of ceiling
light mixing with the fluid. I forced myself to look at the needle and then at Leftwich.

"This is antinomycin. It may make you sick. You'll be getting these shots for the next five days, and you'll probably
have some unpleasant side effects. You probably will lose

your appetite and some weight." He continued to dab my arm with ammonia.

"You will vomit a lot, get the chills . . . you know . . . one of the more severe side effects is that you could lose your hair, and you could get acne."

Dr. Leftwich brought the syringe up and leaned forward to administer the injection. I was faster, jerking my arm away and pulling the rubber tourniquet up, ripping it off my upper arm, my forearm just missing the point of the needle.

CHAPTER FIVE

"Wait a second. I think we should talk to my dad first."
Dr. Leftwich looked surprised and almost dropped the needle. He set the syringe back on the tray, placing it back on the
vanity where it was less threatening.

"Yes, we will, Tom. I'll give your dad a call." Leftwich
was searching for something else to say, but never saying
anything about the biopsy or the other tests. "We need to get
this started. We can't wait."

The side effects he was talking about were frightening.
What was going on? Nobody had ever said anything about
this. Just when was all this going to stop? Another couple of
days here, another couple of days there—and I just kept letting them do it.

"All . . . all right. What's the next step?"

"We'll be giving you these shots for the next five days.
You'll be taking more tests." Leftwich turned and placed the
shot tray back on my bed, bending over to pick up the tourniquet from the floor. The antinomycin would be injected, undiluted, directly into my bloodstream, and I couldn't believe I
was actually letting him go through with it. One part of me
said no, but he was the doctor and supposedly knew what
was best.

"Relax, Tom," he said as he inserted the needle into the
skin, the ugly liquid draining into my arm.

The drug had a peculiar stench, worse than the hospital
smell I had grown to dislike; it was unnatural to have this put

into my body. It took two minutes for the liquid to drain down to a murky pool, following the tiny, thin point of the needle deep into me.

"There we go. All done." Leftwich busied himself with the tray and backed out of the room. Five days of this would put me way back in practice. It was going to be tough catching up with school work, so I closed my eyes, not wanting to worry about it in the early afternoon. Every time I saw Leftwich, it was always bad news.

I was asleep for only a couple of hours and woke up with a fever. I did not want to get out of bed and remembered vaguely talking to a nurse in my room. She talked about Jesus, but I told her I just wanted to be left alone.

The tests were done for the day, but the nausea grew within me as I held my stomach and doubled up in bed, the sickness crawling up my chest and lodging in the back of my throat. I shook with the chills from whatever Leftwich had injected. My pajamas were bunched up around me, wet with sweat.

I thought about God, saying aloud, "Oh, God, it's not going to be like it was before . . . like if I scored a touchdown or did OK on a test . . . you know . . . like when I said I'd go to church and all. I'm not going to say . . . well, I'm just being honest with you. I'm not saying I will go to church, but I am sincere. I'm . . ." I moved to a more comfortable position as I held my eyes tightly closed.

"Lord, I'm not going to promise you I'll go to church every Sunday. I want to be honest with you. Please help me through whatever this is. I'm sorry for the bad stuff I ever did before . . . I will be honest." I found myself reaching out, pawing at the open air.

Sleep was a welcome escape, and it was nightfall when I opened my eyes. It was uncomfortable to lie so still, my skin clammy, cold, and moistened with sweat. I stayed awake the rest of the night.

I got out of bed, squinting as I made my way down the

hall, feeling like I was a Hanoi POW, the blue pajamas drawn tightly around my waist, the sleeves too short and barely reaching my forearms. The light from the nurses' station seemed to follow the fresh slits in my feet, and I almost bumped into two nurses who were walking down the short shaft from the kitchen.

"Well, hello. It walks," they said, almost together, surprised to see me awake.

"I couldn't sleep. After that doctor comes in the morning, I'm going to feel terrible again." I didn't know why I responded that way; maybe because they seemed genuinely interested.

The sutures were taken out in the morning, and my abdominal bandages were removed and replaced with smaller fresh ones. Dr. Leftwich said he'd be in touch with Dad and didn't say much of anything else. He wasn't an altogether unpleasant man, but his conversations with me always delayed my adieu to the hospital. There was always something else—another test, more days of treatment and injections, the seriousness of his voice. I slept for a few hours after he left, awakening nauseous again and sick with dry heaves, finally throwing up in the bathroom. I hadn't taken anything but a betadine shower since the night before leaving the Academy, and my skin was dry, my hair oily, and sweat and the odor of previous days coated my body. The simple task of taking a shower, now that the bandages were removed, was going to be the highlight of my stay.

The water spray hit me directly in the face, the pellets rinsing my hair and rolling down my back. I felt as if I'd jumped into a clear, cold pool on a hot summer's day. The hospital soap made excellent lather, the suds clinging to me, and I washed twice and then again, standing lazily under the nozzle for several moments, the soap suds making swirls around the ceramic tile and gurgling away down the drain. I had to hold on to the vertical, two-foot-long stainless steel bar attached midway up the shower wall. My God, was I weak! My muscles felt flabby, and it was difficult to stand.

I lowered the cover to the commode, sat on it, and gingerly dried my toes, spending almost an hour in the little bathroom. I was sure Navy would do well against Syracuse the next day, and I had to get back in shape. I'd missed a full week of class now, and it would take at least a couple of weekends to catch up. I had to get back to the Academy, back to playing football, and maybe these goals shielded me from everything the hospital was doing. Bethesda was just another obstacle, and I thought then that chemotherapy was just another hospital procedure. I was too naive.

Mary Beth, my oldest sister, was one of the most respected nurses at Saint Joseph's Hospital in Milwaukee, Wisconsin. Mom and Dad had been talking with her often, ever since Coach Welsh had first spoken to Richard, and she decided to come to Bethesda after hearing about the biopsy results. I didn't know it then, but further surgery was scheduled in a few days.

I was awake when she walked into the room. I grinned spontaneously and rose up from the bed, reaching out and extending both arms to draw my sister to me. Our family is close, but we rarely expressed emotion physically—I didn't remember ever hugging her before. It was a strange yet wonderful feeling, and I was happy she was here. Maybe subconsciously I was afraid I wouldn't be leaving the hospital for a while, and, if so, it was nice to have Mary Beth there. She knew what was going on.

Mary Beth didn't say much at first as I complained about looking pale and being weak all the time. I wasn't eating much, and she would watch me grow weaker throughout her visit.

"Tommy, why don't you rest and I'll be right back, OK? I'll be out in the hall for a few minutes." She kissed me on the forehead and walked out to the hallway.

A nurse was seated at the ward station, absorbed with forms and records, paperwork spread out over the red formica of the lower cabinet in front of her.

"Hello. My name is Mary Beth Petersen. My brother is Tom Harper, the midshipman."

The nurse smiled and responded kindly, "Your brother's been taking this pretty well. He hasn't been any trouble. I know he wants to get out of here. It's too bad, you know, he won't be playing football again . . . he's cute."

"Thank you. It looks like you have a good hospital here. I think he's in good hands, and, by the way, I think he'll figure out some way to play."

The nurse nodded in acknowledgment and let my sister review my charts. Mary Beth didn't say anything about them when she came back into my room.

The nurse continued to busy herself with the files in front of her, reviewing comments and routinely doing administrative chores, stopping when her notes showed the template of "Harper, Thomas J., MIDN/USN" embossed on the bottom. The corpsman on duty late the previous night had written about a conversation I'd had with him:

> Patient stated, "Things look as though my life depends on medicine that will change my appearance and probably the way I have lived for 19 years. What other bad news could I possibly get?"

The next entry said:

> This patient should get the very best in spirit-lifting nursing care. With help from the chaplain and help from the staff of T–11, Mr. Harper's depression hopefully can be short-lived.

I wondered how people would feel about me. The medicine was going to make me look terrible—I'd be skinny and pale. I didn't want to show these feelings to anybody and even tried to deny them to myself. I always tried to be in good spirits. What was I going to do? What the corpsman had written didn't really surprise anybody. I was supposed to die.

Mary Beth stayed with me most of the day. Sandra Welsh called that afternoon to say hello, and after chatting with Mary Beth she spoke quietly with me.

"You know, Tommy, I've been going through some of

the coaches' notes about the players and all. You've got a lot
of good stuff written about you. Says here you're probably the
best athlete on the team." Sandra's voice was gentle and soft,
and it was relaxing to listen to her and see my older sister
patiently sitting and smiling at me. I knew Sandra didn't have
any notes in front of her; she was just trying to make me feel
better—and she did.

I refused lunch and turned down another injection, for
nausea, although I did take some medication for a headache.
It would be only a few more hours until the antinomycin
made me sick again, and I couldn't take all the injections,
praying that Leftwich's five-day program would stop. I didn't
need anything else in my body. I wouldn't tell my sister about
the dry heaves and restless nights, hadn't mentioned it to
anyone else, and never would.

Mary Beth wheeled me to more tests, the chest x ray taking longer than normal, and I had another liver scan. My cancer was embryonal cell carcinoma of the testes, with
seminoma. Metastasis was pronounced, and most of my tests
were positive. Simply put, I had testicular cancer, and it was
spreading throughout my body. They had started initial chemotherapy and were looking to see just how far it had spread.
The doctors would split me open down the middle and remove any cancerous tissue—lymph nodes, perhaps carriers of
the disease.

The doctors finished with the tomogram, spending extra
time with the x rays, and Mary Beth and I went to Leftwich's
office together. Dr. Timmons brought in more papers, x rays,
and charts.

Leftwich was direct and to the point. "Tom, the disease
has spread to your lungs—all throughout your lungs. It's
gone farther than we expected. Of course, additional surgery
is out of the question for now." The x rays Dr. Timmons held
looked as if someone had blasted my lungs with a shotgun
full of quarter-sized tumors.

"The news keeps getting worse," was all I could say,
shrugging and looking at my sister, who gently held my
hand. I could tell she was worried about something, but there

wasn't anything I could do to make her feel better. I'd be in the hospital even longer now, but I was happy the next operation had been canceled, since my body wouldn't be marked up anymore. They wouldn't have to split my chest open, and maybe that meant there was a good chance I'd get back to the Academy soon. I didn't know that the surgery had been intended to stop the disease from reaching my lungs. The cancer was already there.

I didn't eat much and wasn't feeling well, illness eating at my belly, but I couldn't let it show. Some Academy people came by, and I tried to act like nothing was wrong. Finally, they were on their way, and Mary Beth was the last to go. She smiled, knowing how badly I felt, and smoothed my hair before she left.

I got out of bed and went into the bathroom, locking both doors and vomiting violently into the toilet, feeling some relief at first, but then the dry heaves came back again, putting me on my knees. I had never been so weak. The light on the bathroom ceiling reflected off the mirror and covered all the cracks in the floor as I shivered and retched until past midnight, the black lid of the toilet seat round and soulless in my hands. I left my room early the next morning for the nurses' station and said to the corpsman on duty, "Let's see what they have to say about me."

"Well, I guess it's OK. Here's your chart."

The corpsman pulled a metal folder from a stack of about 15 others, and I looked over its contents carefully, not paying much attention to the description of injections and test results. I found it under the nursing notes:

> Patient has no complaints. . . . Patient slept most of the shift. . . . Patient spent most of night comfortably.

The words were directly opposite to what had happened the night before. There was a long paragraph about depression, probably entered after the initial antinomycin injection. It was very important, to me, for them not to know how I really felt. I needed to be more careful.

Academy people always came by to see me. I got calls from family and friends and plenty of mail. My sister Jackie mailed a funny card every day, and Admiral Mack, the Academy superintendent, came by while I slept. When they left, I'd catch myself reaching out to them, pawing again at the air, never expecting something like this to happen.

The next few days had a routine about them. Mary Beth would be in my room about 10:30 A.M., just after I'd received my chemotherapy injections. I'd sleep intermittently afterwards, waking up to excuse myself and go into the bathroom, locking the door and retching, mostly in dry heaves. Nurses came and went with the medication. I felt badly about getting sick with Mary Beth there, and a couple of times I didn't make it to the safety of the bathroom and threw up in the wastebasket. I hoped she wasn't telling too many people.

I was supposed to die. The cancer was eating away at my insides, spreading, my chest x rays such that some doctors were surprised I hadn't already asphyxiated. What bothered me most, though, was that I was losing weight. I was a vain jock and didn't know I was supposed to die. I remembered standing in line during Plebe Summer clothing issue, behind my NAPSter friend Steve Barnett, who was a good track and field athlete. People handing out uniforms would stop and look when we gave our size 18 neck measurements, but I became irritated that they'd always ask Steve if he played football and not me. He'd say no, and I'd move forward in the line, chest out, expecting them to ask, but they never would. After a while, I would jump in and say, "This guy ahead of me doesn't play football, but I do!"

Mary Beth gave me a rubdown one day and remarked about how big my back muscles were. I was proud of my physique and told her about lifting weights, working out until my fingers were swollen and every muscle cried out for rest. I couldn't help but think of Captain Sinke. I'd had the duty watch one night during the early spring at NAPS and had decided to lift weights while assigned on tour. I had been devotedly working out five or six hours a day, my interest becoming a religion because I wanted to be Navy's starting tight end for the 1973 season. It was 3:00 A.M., and I was the duty midshipman candidate, in my underwear, pumping iron in the small Tome Inn weight room away from my upstairs duty post. If anybody on campus was awake, I didn't know about it, and at that hour I really didn't care. I hadn't counted on Captain Ralph Sinke having the officer duty, being awake, alive, and wandering the halls.

"Who's the duty? Where's the duty candidate?" They could have heard him bellowing all the way up in Canada.

I was halfway through a lift, but suddenly halted, mumbling to myself, "Oh, shit, it's Captain Sinke." He stood in the doorway of the weight room, hands on hips, the glare of the single fluorescent light reflecting off the summit of his shaved head and rolling down to his effervescent shoes. It wasn't even dawn yet, and Sinke looked exactly as he would for a formal noon inspection. Captain Ralph Sinke was all Marine, from his shaved head to the uniform crease line that ran from his immaculate shirt to pressed trousers and down to those brightly reflective shoe tops.

"What are you doing down here, Harper? What the hell are you doing down here? Where's the duty candidate?"

I stood in front of him, holding a barbell in one hand and trying to keep my boxer shorts up with the other, feeling completely asinine.

"As you know, Captain Sinke, Sir . . ."

"I am not a you, Candidate Harper! The accepted practice of a midshipman candidate is always to address commissioned officers in the third person!"

"Yes, Sir, Captain Sinke, Sir. I am the duty candidate."

The Fox, as we called him, knew what I was doing. I had the duty, there was nothing else to do, and I couldn't sleep, so why not get in an extra workout? Sinke gave me his "you worthless candidate" look.

"Oh, goddamn, goddamn. What the hell are you doing? Get your uniform back on and man your post!"

I was lucky I wasn't restricted for months for having left my sworn duty post.

I'd have done anything to work out back then, and now something was taking it all away. I was always sleepy, tired, and achy like after a brutal football game, not eating much because it was hard to hold anything down. The information was getting worse—the cancer was in my liver, lungs, and spleen, and was blocking some of the channels to my heart.

My parents had been talking daily with the Bethesda doctors and Mary Beth. The hospital had a family lodge, which the Academy reserved for them, and they knew it was time to be with me when test after test after test came back with bad news. I was looking forward to seeing them but I felt apprehensive about it because I had lost so much weight.

Ken McElroy even brought Susie to see me, all the way from Michigan.

"Susie, don't expect it to be the same as before," Ken had told her, as they stopped right before they got to my room. The door to 1119 was open, but they were at the far side of the hall where they couldn't be seen.

"Susie, be strong for Tom. He needs to see you strong," Mr. McElroy said, taking his daughter's hand into his own.

Susie seemed scared at first. I was alone in the room, worn, tired, and gaunt, no sparkle in my eyes. My skin was pale and yellowish.

"Hi, Susie," I managed to say as we hugged each other. We had become good friends.

"I'm sorry . . . sorry I screwed up the weekend. I guess things won't be the same, huh? Jees . . . I never pictured this. I feel like . . ." I stopped. I didn't think Susie understood, and I was too embarrassed to tell her anything.

"I feel like a 90-year-old man."

"It's not your fault, Tommy. I . . . how do you feel? Are you eating OK?"

"Yeah . . . you know, I don't care what they do to me, Susie. I'll be out of here. I'm not about to do this forever, I tell you. I need to work out. I haven't studied in over a week. This is all . . . this is all bullshit." I felt terrible that anyone had to see me like this and confused that everything had gotten so complicated.

"God will work things out, Susie," Mr. McElroy said to his daughter after they left. "You were strong for Tom."

I got liberty over the weekend, going outside for the first time in over a week with Mary Beth and my parents. The initial chemotherapy was over, and there would be no more tests for a couple of days. We rode the elevator down to the hospital rotunda, turning left to go down the hall, and outside across the parking lot toward the guest lodge. I walked, free of the wheelchair, slowly and weakly—but I walked. Dad pushed open the right side of the double doors leading outside, and I motioned Mom and Mary Beth to go first. It was a beautiful day, the air was crisp, and I anxiously anticipated the rush of freshness into my lungs.

I followed them out, but suddenly everything was white and harsh and painful. I became dizzy, wavered, and for an instant that sickening nausea again hit my stomach. Dad grabbed me before I fell down the stairs leading to the parking lot.

"Tommy, are you all right?" I paused for a moment, covering my eyes with my hands and steadying my balance by leaning up against my father. Slowly, I opened my eyes as the outside light filtered through, giving me time to adjust to the new daylight.

"Yeah, yeah . . . I'm OK."

It was an enjoyable weekend, Mom and Mary Beth cooking my favorite meals as we all relaxed and lounged around, free from the chemotherapy. I felt secure, having my parents and Mary Beth with me. Everything would turn out all right—it had to.

Dad spoke with Admiral Mack, but I was asleep when the Academy superintendent stopped by. He had gone out of his way to visit, and my parents were moved by the admiral's personal concern.

"How's Tom?" he'd asked.

"He seems to be doing OK, Admiral. Thank you for what

you and the Academy are doing for him. Coach Welsh and his charming wife have spoken highly of your assistance," Dad replied.

The regulations stated that I would probably have to be discharged from the Academy, but the superintendent didn't talk about that with my parents. He wasn't about to give up on me.

"This is a good hospital, Jack. If there's any way to find a cure, this place will find it—if that young man doesn't find it first himself."

CHAPTER SIX

My parents spent five days at Bethesda; time passed quickly at the lodge. Mary Beth broiled six expensive filets while Mom and Dad mixed fresh vegetables, piling my plate high with a delicious salad. The little kitchenette was filled every day with the aroma of my favorite foods. The grounds outside were manicured and pleasing to stroll, the weather ideal, the sky always blue with daylight and clear with the night stars. The temperature was invigorating, and the crispness of the wind was a pleasant antidote to any dismay they might have felt about my cancer.

I was the fifth of eight children, and whenever any one of my brothers or sisters called it made me feel as if our whole family was together again. The five girls and three boys in our family experienced an energetic, enthusiastic life while we were being raised. Our favorite time of the year as kids was Christmas Day, when we sat around the tree—or trees, since sometimes there were two—taking turns selecting gifts. Everybody had to watch as each present from the residue of Santa's pack was devoured amongst sounds of glee.

Mom and Dad required good behavior, had strict moral principles we all were encouraged to follow, and made considerable personal sacrifices in order to give us good educations and a comfortable, warm place to live. They were charismatic, in a quiet, reserved, peaceful sort of way, strict without being too forceful, loving without being overbearing. We learned that life was valuable—too short to be wasted and too precious to be taken for granted. Our house was a support structure, and from it came faith and the belief that everyone should make a contribution in their lives, to better themselves and their fellow people. I didn't realize then that the outlook on life they passed on to me would have just as great an effect on cancer as any drug or radiation treatment.

Mary Beth kept everyone in the family advised about all the tests, knowing it particularly helped Mom, who felt assured that someone she trusted understood what was really going on. She often had to repeat the same story three or four times a day. Her voice was calm and reassuring, but it was difficult for her to carry on with the impression that I was doing all right, that I was getting better, that things were as normal as they could be. I think my brothers and sisters understood this, and I knew they gave me their moral support and prayers. It wasn't easy to talk in good spirits sometimes. The disease was rampant in my lungs and in my lymph system, but as yet I still didn't know what I really had. Mary Beth didn't think I would live, a thought she never openly expressed until she went home and shared her feelings with her husband.

My older sister had been at Bethesda for more than a week and had gone to Mass at the Academy chapel with my tight end coach, Commander Earle Smith and his family, before Mom and Dad arrived. The voices of the choir floated softly beneath the stained glass as they walked inside, the sound of young voices harmonious and peaceful. What would she tell everybody if I died? It was very difficult and unpleasant for her to think about, especially in the chapel. It only happens to other people, to other families. Tragedy will not strike the Harpers, because there was an invisible shield between us and the rest of the world. But that was not to be, which never seemed so ironic and so painfully real to Mary Beth as on that Sunday in the chapel. My God, she thought, Tom is not going to be a part of this. She left Mass early to walk outside alone.

I had visitors almost every day. Mids came by, football players, close teammates, and coaches, Academy officers, and staff. Several players stayed for a few hours, waiting patiently for me to finish a test or recover from the drugs. The support from the Academy was becoming as important to me, and to Mary Beth and my parents, as the caliber of care Bethesda afforded. I shared in the conversations and show of concern with delight and felt peaceful after everybody left, good thoughts soothing me to sleep.

Captain Sinke marched in one afternoon, immaculate as usual in his uniform, the red stripe down the side of his perfectly cut trousers accentuating his bald head. His shoes were just as spit-shined, his uniform just as creased, as he came in and sat in the chair at the foot of my bed.

"Goddamn, goddamn, Harper. You were going to be my All-American."

I couldn't think of a word to say as Sinke shook his head, never looking at me or at least not into my eyes.

"Well, we finally meet the immortal." My father's voice filled the room, and Captain Sinke jumped up to shake hands.

"Don't believe everything you hear, Sir," Sinke replied.

"I appreciate what you've done for Tom at NAPS. He speaks very highly of you."

"Well, Mr. Harper, you know how young men are these days."

I felt awkward with the Marine captain in the room, and my parents were a welcome relief. I had a different impression of Captain Sinke when he finally left—I didn't see the Vietnam hero, the small college All-American, the officer who'd put his lips a half-inch from my ear and shout commands. I respected that Marine captain, and though my disease seemed a barrier of some kind between us, I was grateful for what he had taught me. I never saw him again.

Being from a large family, when I left to go anywhere I always thought, what's happening with everybody else? All this concern, the stay in the hospital, the reaction to the injections—something wasn't as it should be. I always hoped that nothing serious would ever happen to my brothers and sisters or to my parents, and if whatever this was had to happen to anybody in my family, I was somehow glad it had happened to me. It was my natural reaction and not something egotistical, because to watch someone else suffer was harder than going through it myself. I couldn't deliberate on the tests, the terrible smell of the drugs, or the concern of my family and friends, because I wanted to get on with the next step and establish a routine that would get me out of the hospital. I didn't want to think about getting sick again and didn't understand cancer, not recognizing what a malignant tumor really was. I was told, but didn't want to know what it meant. I couldn't interrupt thoughts of getting well with full consideration of what was wrong with me. It just didn't make any sense. I was still in the hospital, getting rapidly out of shape, and no one seemed interested in telling me when I could expect to leave. It was a Navy hospital, and I was a plebe, and quite possibly I was still enough in awe of the system to do everything they told me. They hadn't said I could leave the hospital, so I stayed.

My parents didn't talk with me about cancer, and I, in turn, never mentioned it. It was obvious the drug treatments were of considerable discomfort, and Mom and Dad were not that unfamiliar with the disease—nor were they strangers to the anxiety of having one of their children ill. It was the finality of cancer, the aura of malignancy and confirmed spread of tumors throughout my body, that concerned them. They had raised eight children—two were married and on their own, three were away at college, two were in high school, and one was in the hospital. There were the usual growing-up crises that always seemed to be solved by their soothing voices and steady hands, but cancer was foreign, a catastrophe they only read and heard about. Death had never stalked their grown family so closely. Their eight children had developed their own personalities, and they had grown with them, living their likes and dislikes, sharing their victories and defeats, anticipating joy and suffering adolescent sorrows. There was always something tangible to fall back on and something they could always do, but my cancer was a will-o'-the-wisp to grasp, elusive to any efforts.

The news wasn't getting any better, although the doctors were positive and cooperative and the facility was ideal. Testicular cancer is typically a young man's disease, and a military hospital like Bethesda would experience more of it because of the relatively young age of men in the U.S. military. The relatively larger number of Bethesda cases, though actually infrequent, had resulted in this hospital having the best treatment available. The spread of this cancer, though, would have made it all hopeless had it not been for my family's deep faith, the support of the Academy, and, at the time, my self-centered attitude toward life—the Naval Academy and football, in particular.

We all went to the Air Force game, where I was given the game ball from the Syracuse contest of the week before, the locker room in pandemonium as everybody celebrated the 49-to-6 Navy victory over the Falcons.

I felt a little awkward and out of place walking down to see the team; my hair was longer than that allowed for a midshipman, and I sported the initial evidence of a moustache. "Hey, he's a recruit. Check the 'stache," somebody said as my teammates crowded around me and rubbed my hair.

Dr. Eichelberger met my parents in the parking lot and was as optimistic as he could be, maintaining a constant level of hope and leaving the door open for change.

Mary Beth and my parents couldn't stay on the East Coast indefinitely, and although they were confident that I was in the right place, it was hard for them to leave without a confirmed cure. I would miss them, but I had to get on with it, all of us knowing I wouldn't be alone.

Dad brought along a simple, old, and well-used brown rosary, pressing it into my palm as they said goodbye. "I want you to have this. It's . . . very special. It's gotten me through a lot of things." I smiled at him. It was an uneasy feeling to see them and my sister leave.

Chemotherapy treatment began again the next Monday, Dr. Timmons occasionally administering the drugs. Mids with terminal disease would lose their position at the Academy, but initially he never addressed that eventuality with me, and I did not bring it up or think about it at first.

My body was changing in a way I could not understand. I was uncommonly tired and slept more, but not as soundly, always wanting to rest and frequently not recalling what people said, who said it, and even what I had just read. I was pale, couldn't hide the pallor, and used makeup with the acne, but it didn't work.

It had come just as Leftwich promised, starting slowly, then rapidly covering my face and chest, puffy white sores and capsulated white pus maturing on my upper body. I applied medication to no avail. Dad had lent me his electric shaver, but I didn't dare shave and couldn't date, looking like this, recalling friends with acne I had felt sorry for in high school—but they never looked this bad. No one said anything directly about my appearance, but in my room I held covers up to my face, not knowing how long I would have to keep to myself.

I was given new drugs and results of the new dosage devastated my body. I had no energy, my muscles felt like jelly, I couldn't eat, and what I finally did eat I regurgitated. I was determined, however, never to show my nausea or vomiting, checking my chart every day to see that the entries were what I wanted:

Patient slept soundly. No complaints.

I left for a new room on the fourteenth floor, tower 14, on Wednesday, October 17. Its bathroom, now my favorite room, was slightly larger but similar to 1119.

The ceramic tile floor was hard and cold, and the light above the sink attracted a moth now and then, a breeze occasionally giving me the chills by sneaking past the crack in the window. I threw up into the bathtub and saved the toilet for the other end—it was too difficult at times to make it either way. I had no strength. I had lifted weights for months, I had run and done well in practice, I was 225 pounds when I came into this hospital, and now I slumped over the commode, pounding the sides with my fists and puking my guts out. It dripped off the sides, and I could feel the slimy and offensive liquid all over my skin where I slouched on the floor, grasping the rim of the bowl with both hands. I closed my eyes and dropped my chin on the lid, exhausted as I tried to catch my breath. The lid of the toilet fell down on my head. Jesus Christ, I thought, what next? I laughed—it was all I could do.

I kept going here, there, and everywhere for tests and more tests. I lost track of the x rays. I grew tired of the bone scans. I didn't like wheelchairs and hated the halls of the ward. I needed to work out and wanted to run, but I didn't have enough energy to make it down the stairs. Something was wrong. Dr. Eichelberger lived close to Dr. Bruce Ruppenthal, a young physician assigned to the small Academy hospital. Ruppenthal and Eichelberger were both close to a Marine lieutenant colonel, assigned to the Academy staff, who had died suddenly after complaining of headaches, abdominal pain, and groin difficulties only 24 hours before. He was admitted to the hospital for overnight observation and tests but was dead before dawn. The autopsy read that testicular cancer had spread to his lungs and throughout his body to the brain. Dr. Ruppenthal received word only a couple of days later that the midshipman Dr. Eichelberger had sent to Bethesda had this same disease, and it was ironic to him that they had a healthy Marine officer who died suddenly from it and now a midshipman whose prognosis was equally grim.

No one told me this. Dr. Eichelberger would have told me I had cancer, but I never asked him. My swollen testicle was an external symptom, but the lieutenant colonel had nothing, no external warning signal until considerable discomfort set in at the end. God worked in strange ways to Marty Eichelberger—everything and everyone had a purpose. A surgeon, an individual, a family—many times they could only do so much, and the rest was best left to God's will. I wasn't incapable of understanding that and wanted to be aware of life, not wanting to dwell on anything else. God had helped me out before, and I always thanked him, knowing all I had to do was ask, which I did. I had to get back to the Naval Academy and to my football team.

Dr. Elliott Perlin had served as head of Bethesda's oncology department for more than seven years, a career Navy physician, slight of frame and balding with a gray speckled beard, a man fascinated by malignancies and the work toward successful treatments, and a doctor highly respected by his contemporaries. He was asked to make recommendations regarding my care and came to the ward to examine me, concurring with the diagnosis of advanced testicular cancer after reviewing the pathology exam, which showed embryonal cell cancer. He knew testicular cancer accounted for a good percentage of deaths in young men, and he measured certain proteins in my blood which reflected a significant activity of the disease.

My diagnosis was incurable in the 1960s; chances in 1973 were a little better, although less than 10 percent. Dr. Perlin, however, never played numbers with me, telling me just what they were going to do and that we'd be a team. Dr. Leftwich had done his job, and I did not see him again, but I was grateful, I guess, for what he had done. Dr. Perlin was now responsible for my care, advising Dr. Timmons and Dr. Grady on the floor, and if a decision was made it was made on his advice.

Dr. Perlin initiated a program of chemotherapy and radiation; the radiation was experimental and based upon medical literature that suggested then that there was a better effect if the whole lung was subjected to radiation and the areas of tumor involvement were boosted with extra x rays. He knew my lungs could be affected permanently, that I would have impaired breathing capacity, but it had to be done and I was prepared to do anything to get out of that hospital. The football season was already half over.

The walk to radiation was dismal and smelled of burning flesh, the place in the bowels of Bethesda. I wore the same blue POW pajamas—loose because I'd lost so much weight—going down the hallway where the little boy and I had had the wheelchair races, walking past the post office, down by the pharmacy waiting room, and past the out-patient clinic.

The double doors near the hospital chapel were a bother, the door on the left always locked, the one on the right always difficult to open as I spoke aloud, "What a pain in the ass."

The first time I took radiation, I thought, My God, they've sent me by the chapel, but I made it a habit to stop inside going to and from each treatment. It was quiet there. I'd sit in a pew for a few minutes, recite an Our Father and Hail Mary, before honestly and simply praying to God. I just asked him to help me get out of the hospital. I'd sit in a front row pew if no one else was around, always entering through the same door and picking the very last pew if anyone else was there. It was quiet and peaceful, the light blue color of the carpet complementing the soft brown brick, covered by recessed lighting. Wooden slats rose vertically to meet the light fixtures and gave support like churches everywhere to the large crucifix behind the altar. I used to stare at the cross, and it seemed as if his head moved as I glanced back and forth, looking up from reading the religious literature I'd picked up from the back of the chapel. Time was slow, relaxed, and it was easier to think there about the happy events of my life and to reflect on what the future held in store. No matter what happened on a particular day, I always left there in a peaceful state of mind.

The small corridor past the chapel had a stuffiness that carried peculiar body smells. Loose furniture was on the right side of the hall—rusty stuff, covered with grime—and old, broken chairs half-heartedly leaned against the musty corridor wall. Not much, if any, light came through the dirty, dusty windows, hiding all the color except the green of a large door at the end of the corridor that proclaimed, "Radiation Waiting Room."

I pushed it open and ran my hand along the greenish yellow tile that led to therapy. The waiting room was a dismal place, its floor covered by a faded brown carpet and rows of crumbled plastic chairs above which hung nondescript pictures of Navy ships. The walls were pink and outlined in dirty orange trim, and there was a yellowed, hand-written note, crookedly hung by a locked door, which proclaimed, "All Patients Waiting—moderate to excessive lapsed time awaiting treatment . . .," the rest of the verbiage claiming the harassment of the harried corpsmen and a request for patience. It was annoying.

I had to walk down eight steps to get inside the actual treatment room, the walkway leveling off for three feet, then going down further between heavy steel railings. A glass-enclosed technician's booth looked down on everything in the chamber.

I hated this room; it was like a large grave, sealed behind a massive four-inch-thick steel door, which was bolted down to heavy runners, wide valves running along its edge at eye level and up into the wall above. The door was open when I arrived, and I would lay naked on the cold slab, beneath an evil-looking machine that hovered above me like a giant mosquito. Lead markers were placed on my stomach, and other ingots were positioned where the doctors didn't want me subject to radiation. They painted red lines from my neck to the lower part of my stomach, like an alleyway, with the ingots outside the lines. The door would slowly roll to a close, and a permanent clunk echoed throughout the chamber, closing me inside, alone. I never liked that feeling. It was depressing, and it gave me the creeps; the atmosphere was one of defeat and termination. I did it only because it was part of the therapy I was told to take. I prayed under that mechanism, beseeching the Lord through repeated pronunciations of the Our Father and Hail Mary, trying to defeat the feelings of dread the machine induced as it did its work.

The radiation therapy itself didn't hurt, but shortly after the treatments started I found it hard to breathe. I tried to run again, several times, and the radiologist would tell me not to try running anymore.

"Do you realize how close you are?" he said, mad because I had been on him about running for two days.

"I've got to run. I'm playing football. I've got to run and get in heavy with the weights. Can't you get me off this?"

The radiation was getting to me, and I had to find a way to let out my frustration. The doctor was visibly angry.

"You're not going to play football again! Forget that! Don't you realize what's wrong with you? How serious you are?"

I didn't say anything to him after he finished yelling, and he just shook his head and made a few scribbles in my chart. Couldn't he see that, no matter what, I had to concentrate on getting back into shape? I didn't care what his opinion was about running or my condition. I had to keep my sights completely aimed at getting back into shape. There could be no distractions.

I still tried to run, forgetting the radiologist's opinion, but I couldn't. It hadn't been that long since I beat Dr. McCaffery, a friendly, outgoing man who sometimes helped with my chemotherapy, in basketball, telling him as he administered the drugs, "I know why you're giving me this now—so you can kick my ass in basketball."

He laughed, his sense of humor temporarily hiding the sickening feeling of the drugs going into me. It had only been a couple of days, but the basketball game with McCaffery seemed like it was years ago as I lay upon the cold slab for another treatment, radiation scars now all over my chest.

Dr. Timmons had a substitute one day—a short, blond, young doctor who acted as if he was there to pass judgment when I started to talk to him about football.

"Hey, you're not going to make it," he said, looking at me as if he was saying, "You're stupid, kid."

I often walked the grounds of Bethesda alone, leaving my room and going down the elevator or sneaking out slowly down the back stairs. I watched the building of the Mormon Temple, far away behind the beltway, from a manicured rise that overlooked a tree hollow lining the bank of the creek below. It was a quiet setting, and I had to remind myself at times to go back to my room.

I'd go out to the main entrance flagpole occasionally, wearing a bathrobe over the pajamas, the concrete and asphalt hard under my slippers. I watched the ants that ran along the base of the sidewalk by the old ship's mast, and in a way they had things to do and so did I. It had only been September 28 when I had gotten out of the Navy station wagon, stopping over briefly at the hospital here, en route to play against Michigan. I didn't play against Michigan; I hadn't played since; I couldn't run; my muscles felt like marshmallows. What the hell had happened? I had to catch up.

I would make it. I thought about football every day, the Academy and my friends there, my family. I would make it, and besides, I had already asked God. The support of the Academy and the majority of the staff at Bethesda far outweighed any contrary conclusions. Most people who took the time to visit gave me positive reinforcement. The little things added up, regardless of how badly they really felt about my chances, and I could never tell how badly they felt because none of their worry ever came across. It is excellent medicine.

I was doing better than some others in the ward. There was an older gentleman, a retired admiral, who died a little every day—a proud man, still resolute despite the disease which raged within him. We talked a lot, but I mostly listened as he told of his wartime experiences and of past fellow officers now dead, the exploits garnished over the years. He knew he was going to die and resigned himself to that fate. What was inside him would kill him and was something over which he felt he had no control. The old admiral would lie in bed, at times taking an interest in all the newspapers and magazines that cluttered the top of his small, movable vanity. He'd moan during the night, and I tried to help, holding him tightly as he'd cry on my shoulder, waiting to die. I was only a plebe.

I learned about my true condition shortly after the admiral's death. I was going through my chart at the nurses' station after the usual treatment, and as usual I didn't feel well, but it was important to check my written progress. Everything looked OK except for a short note mentioning three to six months, which struck me as unusual. While walking away from the station, I overheard one nurse say to another, "It's really tragic. He's such a good-looking kid. They don't give him but three months or so. Cancer is destroying him."

I stopped in the hall. Cancer? Three months? Three months to what? My charts said three to six months, too. Three months to live? I felt like saying something, but I didn't know all that much about cancer. It had to be all bullshit. But these people were saying that in three months I would be dead. This couldn't happen—I had to get back to the Academy, to the football team, to the Brigade.

The whole thing just didn't seem real. Had I been led

along all this time? Was I really that stupid? Was I going to die here? I was scared and angry and wondered what they would tell me next. They had to be wrong, and I resolved to prove them so.

I started my own routine. No one dared turn on the lights in my room early in the morning. I didn't like breakfast shoved in front of me, so I canceled it. I wasn't sure if they were feeling sorry for me or were just putting up with a kid with an overburdened ego, but it really made no difference. I wasn't going to let cancer control me without a fight, and having my own way about things I could control made a difference. The difficulty was in controlling my reaction to the things I couldn't do anything about. I had to learn to adjust, to continue with a technique that worked, and to discard whatever wasn't working. I was learning to stay involved.

Dr. Timmons and Dr. Grady kept up with the chemotherapy, and I made it a practice to ask permission to work out, by trying to run or lifting weights, but usually just walking, before the injections. They knew I didn't want other people seeing me sick or even knowing about it. Why would I go through the pain of exercise even though I would be reacting to treatment in a more violent fashion? These workouts were motivation, something to make me stay in shape, the hurt a good hurt; I would forget about the nausea, the vomiting, the diarrhea, and the burning lungs; sweat was healthy, and the odor of drugs and the insipid radiation momentarily forgotten.

I had a new problem if I was as sick as everybody said. I would be discharged from the Academy, and then what would I do? Go to some veterans' hospital in California? Hang around my room at home in San Mateo? No longer be a football player? No longer be a midshipman? But maybe I would be dead before it came to all that. Many people seemed to think so. I talked with Dr. Timmons about it, and while he was sympathetic he was also realistic, saying that he hoped nothing like that would happen, but it was a distinct possibility. I mentioned this to Coach Welsh and Commander Smith, and they both said they would help me, but I knew there was only so much effect their influence could have. The

Navy's Bureau of Medicine was faceless to me, and if Admiral Mack couldn't help, I would no longer be a midshipman.

Dr. Perlin and everybody wrestled with how much they could do, to what extent I could receive the different combinations of drugs and radiation, whether I could hack it. They didn't want to hold out any false hope or offer any undue pessimism, and while there were no guarantees, there were always feelings of hope. It was as effective as any drug or radiation therapy could ever be.

I needed that hope after the first three weeks of combined therapy. I was very outgoing before I started the treatment and tried to be friendly with everyone, but one day I didn't want to do anything. I didn't want to talk or work out; I withdrew, lying in bed all day. Dr. Timmons noticed my endurance drop significantly. I was trying to grasp onto something in order to move on—maybe it was only a dream that I could still play football, or even get back into school. Maybe I would die.

"You can just see the frustration in the guy," Timmons said to Dr. Grady, "He can't do it, but he's still trying. I hate to see a man go down like that. He was a bruiser, remember?"

I completed an EEG, a brain scan, after complaining of frequent mental lapses, not remembering whom I had just talked to or what I had just said. I messed up the treatment schedule and didn't know what I'd had to eat, the food often tasteless and dry. They were afraid the cancer was in my brain. I was talking with a nurse, Mary Campbell, and finally said to her, "Mary, I don't have any idea of what you've said for the last 15 minutes."

"Yes, Tom, I know."

I had gone through a lot to get to Annapolis in the first place. I'd made the varsity football team, and there was no way I'd accept leaving the Academy just yet. I wasn't worried about the brain scan or about the treatment and its side effects, or even dying, to the degree that I was worried about getting back to USNA. I told Dr. Timmons, "Push as hard as you can."

Dr. Grady, a Naval Academy graduate himself, told me one afternoon what Dr. Timmons had told him. "John, this scares me. I can relate to this big, strong kid. You can see the cancer, you can see the tumors on the x ray, but, doggone it, you sure can't see it in him."

"Tom," Grady said to me, "if there was ever a person who can beat this, it's you. I know you hate the radiation and the chemo, but you've got a goal—that's the key. You can do it!"

I knew I had too much to lose to give in. My family, the Academy, Bethesda people, the football team, everybody—they were behind me, and I would do the things I didn't like to do in order to get back to the Academy, play football, and graduate. There was no other way.

I lay in bed thinking about that. It was a quiet afternoon, my therapy way over for the day, and I was tired, not really hungry, and wondered how long it would be before I could leave Bethesda. My upper chest felt as if it was falling down to my groin. I was queasy, weak, and as I touched my hands together my fingernails came off. It wasn't painful. They just crumbled softly between the sheets and onto the floor.

CHAPTER SEVEN

The superintendent's house lies in a pretty setting along the east side of the chapel, across a gentle curve around the first wing of Bancroft Hall. A blue and white striped canopy covers the second-story porch that overlooks a manicured, spacious garden, and well-tended plants hide behind high walls. The temperature had been abnormally hot during the fall of 1973, but there was a slow, refreshing briskness in the early evening air. The green grass in front of the house and along the red-bricked, winding paths of Stribling Walk was resplendent, perhaps noticed this time of year by a superintendent who happened to glance out from an upper-story window upon the Yard.

The mansion stayed the same over the years, apparent by the stoic appearance of its granite and ivy-covered facade, though interior accoutrements would change, depending on the life style and taste of the occupants. Superintendents were a different breed, each admiral lending his own style to the brigade of midshipmen and to all those who served the Academy in various capacities.

Admiral Mack had reported for duty in 1972, Annapolis his last tour of duty after 36 years of active naval service. He was committed to upgrade both professional training and the motivation of midshipmen to stay with the program, to graduate and serve with the fleet. Attitude was the essential ingredient, and the admiral felt anyone who passed the entrance requirements possessed those sometimes intangible characteristics needed to graduate. Admiral Mack introduced better

programs for mids to make up failed courses, even if it meant
not graduating with your class, and every effort was made to
assist a midshipman as long as you reciprocated with an honest effort.

The Naval Academy, nevertheless, is not a hospital or a
haven for those with a disease. The Navy is a fighting service,
and those in its commission are required to be healthy and
vigorous. The Navy takes care of its own, certainly, with the
expertise of the Medical Corps, but some people have to be
discharged, with the Veterans' Administration detailed to
handle the convalescence if possible. This was not a heartless
agreement, but a simple statement of mission and purpose, of
which Admiral Mack was acutely aware when news of my
initial therapy reached him. I was in that category, which worried me, as the Naval Academy of 1973 was not a place to go if
you were looking for cancer treatment. I did not want to go to
a VA hospital.

Academy policy dictated that a midshipman would be
discharged from the Navy if a problem developed during the
first three years that could keep you from getting commissioned. Malignant disease was in that bracket, and dismissal
was certain unless a written waiver was accepted. I wondered
what thoughts were going through the mind of the man who
occupied the superintendent's house. He held my fate in his
hands, and though I could face the Bethesda routine on my
own terms, Admiral Mack's decision was almost beyond my
grasp. I did not like to think about the alternatives and concentrated on staying one step ahead of the therapy that was
gradually eroding my body.

Dr. Perlin was cautious, cluing me in on any unpleasant
news with subtle voice inflections and an empathy that
showed in his eyes.

"What's in this chemotherapy that makes me so sick?" I'd
asked. He was pleased I'd brought it up, because he never
really knew how much a particular problem was bothering a
patient unless the patient talked about it.

"Tom," Dr. Perlin replied, "cancer cells are similar to normal healthy cells. Many of the drugs, the chemotherapy we

administer, like the bleomycin you've been getting, have mo-
lecular configurations that can damage the normal cells. One
of the problems we have is to come up with a drug that has
what we call a good therapeutic index, which compares heal-
ing effect to toxicity. In other words, chemotherapy involves
toxic drugs—poison, if you will—to kill the tumors. Healthy
cells are affected. They do suffer. You're going to get . . .
rather unpleasant side effects."

Perlin tried to be positive, no matter how advanced the
disease, and wouldn't set up negative treatment. Dr. Perlin
didn't let the idea of death take control of me—I wouldn't
have let it, anyway. He always said, "What can we do to cure
this patient? Let's be life-aware." New treatments, new drugs,
had come along in the treatment of testicular cancer, and if
used in the right way and promptly there was a chance of
cure. In 1973, however, there were still a great many patients
with my diagnosis who died from the disease.

I was frightened at times, talking with Dr. Perlin, as I
didn't really know what to expect. He didn't tell me what
I didn't need to know, and I saw the picture as it would be
if I didn't respond to treatment. The disease was spreading
rapidly, and Dr. Perlin was concerned about the tumors en-
larging. It was impossible to remove all of the tumors in my
lungs, which was the reason why the surgery had been canceled, my medical record stating, "No node dissection performed because of distant metastasis."

My endurance continued to deteriorate, but I worked
hard at increasing my exercise tolerance. I still couldn't run,
but after what Dr. Perlin told me I was determined to undergo
the treatments, no matter how difficult they were.

A five-day cycle of chemotherapy started, and as I sat in
the blue treatment room one afternoon they broke the news to
me that I'd be doing this chemo cycle for at least two years,
accompanied with radiation therapy for the next couple of
months.

Oh, my God, I thought, I've got to do this for two years?
I heard what they were saying, but I didn't listen, as my mind
was racing to schedule how I would organize football practice

and meet all the games, how I would make up for lost time with my studies and still graduate with the class of 1977. Surely not all this time would be at the hospital—I had to get back to school and to football. I made up my mind to be ready for the 1974 season—not discharged, certainly not incapacitated, but recovered and back as a Navy football player. There were still three good seasons left, and I did not want to spend the next two recovering from the devastating effects of the treatment.

They finally had told me what I had been wondering about for days—what was next, what was the schedule, what I had to do to get out of the hospital—and when they did, my heart sank, my throat went dry, my knees weakened. Two years of chemotherapy at 28-day intervals for five straight days—it seemed like an eternity. I had to be sick for another 700 days, throwing up for two years, acne all over my face for two years, no more jock ideas, total reclusion. I couldn't believe it—more than two years? I had thought about many things in the future but had never seriously planned ahead. I had to do that now, because the chemotherapy forced me to. I was sick for two weeks after every cycle of chemotherapy, and now I had to go through this every month for the next two years. It was an agonizingly slow process to get over those drugs.

I sat in a comfortably padded chair for the chemo, trying to relax as if I were at home, asleep on an overstuffed couch. There were bottles of sterile water on top of the small sink in the treatment room, stainless steel cabinets with medicine behind glass shelves, and pamphlets proclaiming, "Chemotherapy and You" and "For You the Patient." The ceiling lights overhead and the fluorescent fixtures by the sink cast a contrasting hue over the red vial blood samples, the small containers lined up in order for delivery to the lab. A folded wheelchair behind the door was a stark reminder that this was not a physical therapy room for football players or the Bancroft Hall sick bay. It was different, knowing how I'd feel once the treatment was over and seeing other cancer patients, some pale with fatigue, others balking and frustrated by the routine. I had to be active, and if it wasn't by playing football, then it would be by working my way back so that I could play again.

Dr. Perlin's office was down the hall from the chemo room and was a buffer to the routine whenever I was reluctant to go through another treatment. His smooth porcelain collection was a nice contrast to the government-issue furniture of his office, as was the framed Hippocratic oath that hung on the wall. I told him I'd been going to the Edward Stit Library, adjacent to the brass-railed balcony overlooking the hospital rotunda, to read about testicular cancer and the spread of it. Perlin had mixed feelings about patients studying their disease. An informed patient understood the ailment better and might interact positively with the doctor when various things were explained, but when patients lack the sophistication to interpret what they learn accurately, the whole therapy process could be jeopardized. It could leave one with self-doubt, regardless of a doctor's optimism.

There were many rumors that circulated throughout the Academy, NAPS, and even my old high school concerning my Bethesda status. I didn't hear about too many of them until much later; some stories had me castrated, others completely sterile, and a few portrayed me as a one-legged amputee. I needed to keep my outlook positive, and it was important to remind myself of that. The happy voice of Diana Ross gave me needed boosts of motivation when I played my radio in the early afternoon, wearing earphones and listening to her sing, psyching myself to get ready for radiation and chemotherapy. Many times, after a hard workout and a soothing melody, I was in the treatment room with my arm pumped up and saying, "Give me the drugs, give me the drugs." I'd play soft music afterwards, maybe five or six hours later, to ease the nausea. The music therapy was a powerful magic, exercising control over my mind, making me shift from dwelling on what I didn't want to happen to concentrating on the good things ahead.

Two nurses, Mary Campbell and Mary Hillebrand, gave me a great deal of their time and love. Hillebrand was my ideal nurse—a very attractive blonde, with deep blue eyes and a friendly, outgoing personality. She was an outdoors type and thought I had to be a little crazy to handle cancer the way I did. Campbell was a pretty brunette, tall and slim and one of the most conscientious people I'd ever come across. They both were only a few years older than me.

Hillebrand invited me out to dinner once, to the apartment they both shared. I was a little out of it, primarily because I knew Mary Campbell would be there. I didn't want to impose and, besides, I was still a Plebe, so I said no. Shortly thereafter, I received a call from Campbell. "What's wrong with you, Harper?" she exclaimed.

"What?" I responded, immediately embarrassed.

"Jees, you really are sick. Here you bitch and moan about being in the hospital all day. You can't sleep, you can't eat, you can't do this, you can't do that. I don't know. Jees, you midshipmen are weird. Well, are you going to come over, or are you just going to sit there and feel sorry for yourself?"

"Well, I . . ."

"We'll be over in ten minutes to pick you up. Meet us out by the flagpole. Bye."

Hillebrand and Campbell were always positive, never thinking I would actually die from cancer. Maybe I was too self-centered, with my constant dialogue about football and appearance, and maybe my ego wouldn't let me succumb. They knew that. That first night with these two nurses was absolutely great. They fixed me nice, big, juicy hamburgers, my first "real" food in a long time, and when I had my first sip of rum and vodka I nearly fell over. It was something else—stuffing myself and easing it down with good-tasting drinks. I could barely see across the room by the time it was over, but I didn't care. I was with two attractive women, in a nice apartment, oblivious to chemotherapy and radiation and the hospital and tests—and cancer.

I went back as often as I could. We never talked about cancer there. How could I? They didn't want to, and they wouldn't let me. I either had a drink in my hand or was dodging a flying pillow, the fluffy missile immediately lobbed in my direction if they saw even the slightest bit of a frown.

"Tommy, have some more of this," or, "For a football

player, you sure are slow"—their chatter was constant. "You play for Navy? God help us all . . ."

I had to defend my honor somehow.

"If you're so macho, surely you can have another. We'll drive you back. C'mon."

I needed the support and humor of those two girls. There was never a dull moment at their place, and I always looked forward to going there.

I ended up in Georgetown's M Club Bar right before Thanksgiving. I'd had radiation treatment in the morning and slept in for a few hours. There was a Spanish–American War veteran across the hall, the retired ex-Marine captain filling the ward with the cackles of his weathered voice. He was quiet and asleep when I decided to go out to a restaurant on the outskirts of the hospital. I'd been eating more lately and needed a break from the Bethesda menu. After checking the duty roster, I knew leaving wouldn't be a problem, since Mary Campbell had the late-afternoon shift.

I enjoyed leaving the tall, white hospital tower and walked along just looking at other people go about their business and all the cars passing by. The hospital was a lonely place. Though my friends would visit often, they could only stay for a couple of hours or so out of the day. No visitors were allowed late at night or in the early morning, and sleeping during the day kept me awake most of the night. I was depressed many times, but outside the hospital I forgot about my room, the chemotherapy, the radiation chamber, and the daily routine of tests and treatment. It was a totally different world. I still had my hair, one personal luxury that hadn't succumbed like all the others to Dr. Leftwich's warning.

I decided to keep walking as I approached the restaurant. It was still light out, and I had plenty of time, so I proceeded down Wisconsin Avenue, a soft wind at my back which I could feel drifting along the outside of my dark blue Navy peacoat. My acne had cleared up, but I felt a strain all through my legs as I lifted one foot past the other. I strolled past small shops and businesses, people passing me by, kids riding bikes, cutting in and out of all the pedestrian traffic. I didn't say anything to anyone as I wondered about what was going on back at the Academy.

I was automatically marked absent at my last formation before leaving for Bethesda, because of football, by the upper-classmen. We were required to be there for Thursday's noon formal inspection, and I didn't have a fresh haircut—I had wanted to go to the Michigan game with as much hair as possible. They read my name from the roster while going through the ranks, my squad leader answering that I was absent, so I had to thrust out my arm, perpendicular to my chest in the proper plebe manner, and shout, "Sir! But I am present, Sir!" Not many of the upperclassmen in my company knew who I was, dressed in a regular uniform, since usually I was busy with football and always wore nondescript whiteworks. My squad leader knew I was headed for Ann Arbor the next day, and he approached me with three of his classmates. I was thankful to have taken extra care with my inspection uniform, and luckily nobody said anything to me. That was almost two months ago, and I wondered if marking Tom Harper absent was now an accustomed practice back at Bancroft.

There was a mixture of grocery stores and apartments, fast-food places and small bookstores along the way to Georgetown, and I passed movie theaters and banks and small dress shops with no destination in mind. I heard from someone in my family every day, and wondered what everybody else was doing right now, so many miles away. I'd written Richard the day before to let him know I wouldn't lose either my hair or my senses, as my EEG test results were normal.

I passed a large Episcopalian church on the other side of the street, Wisconsin Avenue bending to the left and going downhill. I had been walking for over two hours. I was very tired, but I felt much better than if I'd been lying in bed trying fruitlessly to sleep. I didn't have a tumor anyone could feel, with no visibly swollen lymph nodes or remarkably enlarged liver, and there was nothing anybody could go on other than what the doctors could find in the x rays and test results, such as analyzing various protein levels in my blood. They would pierce my index finger in the chemotherapy room for that. I hated the sharp sting just before the yellowish chemo fluid would drain into my arm. Lesions were all over my body.

Dr. Perlin would increase or decrease the dosage occasionally, and I picked up on when to anticipate it by watching my blood count. Several times it was so low that treatment was canceled, my resistance to infection affected, and on occasion I was restricted to my room, and no one was allowed to enter. Other times I'd get half a dosage, which got me out of the treatment early but still didn't make me feel any better.

I felt chilly as I walked along, slowly passing large houses almost hidden from the road, smoke coming out of their tall chimneys. Cords of wood were stacked here and there, signaling the cooler temperature that came with the late November sun, now resting on the horizon. There was no firmness to my chest, and my stomach muscles were soft, responding weakly when I flexed. My biceps were hidden somewhere in my upper arms, and my wrists looked smaller, attached to hands that were puffy and pale. I kept walking, not really knowing where I was going. I'd been working on an exercise bike back at the Bethesda weight room but I didn't seem to be making any progress whatsoever.

I was wearing the only pants I had, and I stared at the cuffs of my red checkered trousers as they followed my stride back and forth, my skin sweaty and yet cold beneath the peacoat. I'd forgotten how far a distance I'd put between myself and the hospital. Several drivers had their car lights on, and the glare of the street lights and the signs of bars and clubs lent an irregular glow to the early evening and the fading light of dusk. This time of day had always been my favorite. The setting this day was the same, but new circumstances had turned my anticipation into dismay about what I was missing—my friends, football, and the Academy. I had to keep telling myself I was doing OK.

I remembered the M Club from NAPS days, a small, quiet, dark little bar where the proprietor left you alone. The beer was always cold there, and I walked in just as that night's band was warming up, the sound of their instruments clear and striking. I sat by myself at a table to the left side of the bar and ordered a beer. The band started their first number, and I tapped the beat with my right foot, drinking my beer in slow, steady swallows. There was some satisfaction in putting down an empty mug, the frost on its base creating a small, ringed pool of water that reflected the soft light of the showcase floor and the dark rings below my eyes.

I was tired; it was close to 10:00 P.M., and I had walked more than 11 miles. I wasn't about to walk back. I used a pay phone by the entrance to call Bethesda, getting the operator to switch me to the nurses' station on tower 14.

"Mary?" I said.

"Where have you been?" came her concerned reply. "I've been here hours past my shift trying to figure out where you are. You'd better get back."

"I'm not walking," I replied, and explained where I was.

Two corpsmen and a marine picked me up, arriving in a gray Navy van, the corpsmen dressed in white and the Marine wearing combat fatigues. The trio stopped by the bar long enough to have the bartender point me out. Jesus, I thought, people in this place probably think I've escaped from an asylum somewhere. Who's that? What's wrong with him? They're taking him away!

I was cocky with all the doctors and nurses for the week after that journey, challenging them with my full head of hair, and I felt as if I'd achieved a major victory one day when one of them said, "Hey, Tom, it looks like you're not going to lose your hair after all. Looks like you're going to get by."

The next morning there was a ticklish sensation around my nose and cheeks, and with one open eye I could see tiny hairs next to my face on the pillow. It came out in my hands as I touched it—clumps of hair, leaving my skull spotty and misshapen. I had talked a lot with an enlisted sailor who was going through chemotherapy with me and who had lost all of his hair. He was dead now—the only person with whom I could feel comfortable being seen like this.

Other than Hillebrand and Campbell, none of the nurses or corpsmen on the floor thought I would live, and although they never directly let on to that, after being around for so long I could sense how they felt. I didn't begrudge them and concentrated instead on whatever it was that would help me, rather than think about what other people thought. I wouldn't let anyone into my room when I was really sick, preferring the privacy in which to vomit and experience all the other gross things that came with therapy. The staff could hear me getting sick, and it was not easy to negotiate vomit and diarrhea coming from both ends of me and sometimes all over the bathroom floor.

There had always been someone or something to emulate before—someone to imitate, to pattern myself after. Ted Kwalich, the former Penn State All-American, played tight end for the San Francisco 49ers and was my football hero, so I tried to play the game like he did. Captain Sinke was my first role model in the military, so I tried to look as professional in uniform as he did. I appreciated the style of Helen Brewer, my high school English teacher, and I tried to follow her interest in literature. I read many books while in the hospital, even with my comprehension distorted from the drugs, but I could not find any cancer patient to model myself after. Every article and book I read dealt with "Coping with Dying" or "Death and the Cancer Patient" and seemed to tell a story of courage and wrenching treatment, the impact upon patient and family, the constant struggle to find a cure. But the main character usually died—a victim. I could not concentrate on death and did not want to think of dying. But I could find no book that concentrated on a real awareness of what I was going through, that had life as its constant thread and the quality of life at that.

I prayed earnestly to God and had always been answered before, perhaps in ways I could not understand, so I decided to be my own model, to be my own hero, and someday to relate my experience to others to help them better understand and react to the affliction. This was an attitude that might have been described as egotistical, but I learned to temper that partially. I was no evangelist, having continual bouts with depression, self-pity, and fear, but my subconscious was tuned to living. I tried to associate with circumstances that would get me back to where I was before and to discard anything that wouldn't help me get to where I wanted to go. I was a cancer patient, not a victim, and cancer was an interruption of my schedule.

I watched the 1973 Army–Navy game from the basement of my friend Tom Hutchinson's house, just a short drive from Bethesda in nearby Camp Springs, Maryland. The split-level, contemporary house was always open to me, Tom's parents going out of their way to be hospitable. We ate fried chicken, shrimp, and every other conceivable delicacy while watching the game, surrounded by all the sounds and color of the traditional rivalry. The final score was Navy 51, Army 0. The game was dedicated to me at the pep rally the day before, and a large sheet poster with my name on it hung with all the others in the Bancroft Hall rotunda—"Beat Army for Tom Harper," it read, the words intermingled with other portrayals of our supremacy over West Point.

I received several telephone calls during the next few days, everybody from Annapolis calling to cheer me up and telling me not to worry. Worry? Worry about what, I thought? And Phil Nelson finally told me what had happened. An overexuberant cheerleader had grabbed the microphone during the Pep Rally, exclaiming to the excited crowd in front of him that the game was dedicated to Tom Harper, a plebe football player dying of cancer. I had no intention of lending any accuracy to that well-meaning dedication.

I had missed so much of the first semester that it would require several extra hours and courses to catch up. The academic schedule was well on its way toward final exams, and I wondered what would be necessary to guarantee that I'd get back into the regular Academy routine. This uncertainty left a nagging doubt and seemed to be a roadblock to the treatment, yet I was not aware then of Admiral Mack's deep concern and the compassion that was reflective of his entire Navy career. He admired positive spirit, especially motivation supported by real and meaningful acts. I had been in excellent physical condition before my diagnosis and because of that was able to undergo increasingly heavy dosages of chemotherapy and radiation. I made all of my appointments and told anyone who would listen that I'd be getting back to the Academy and would play football again.

Admiral Mack was aware of this, and though he was not visibly involved, he did subtly direct the doctors' opinion to stress admission back into the Naval Academy rather than emphasize that I had a serious problem. I didn't realize the admiral's intent then, or his own background as a Navy tight end more than three decades earlier. I was self-centered, worrying about my own recovery, my status as a midshipman, my status as a football player; but if it was possible to exert willpower over cancer, I certainly tried, and Admiral Mack's help made it all the better.

The Academy hadn't experienced that many cases of midshipmen with tumors, or Hodgkin's disease, or leukemia. They usually didn't keep those with lung metastasis, as there was concern that the tumors would keep somebody from breathing properly. Many times I'd lie in bed after chemotherapy and the slightest rise in another person's voice would ring in my ears. A corpsman told me that 90 percent of the patients he saw survived cancer only to die later because of the treatment. He didn't say anything about me, and I didn't tell him I had tumors throughout my lungs.

I was tempted to be lazy and disheartened. Patients were told so many times they were supposed to be sick, they were supposed to be tired, and thus most of the time they were— myself included. So much of it is mental. I tried once to run up the stairs to my room instead of taking the elevator from the first floor. I stopped on the seventh floor to rest and was awakened two hours later by a doctor, who asked "What are you doing here?"

"Oh. I'm supposed to be on tower 14." I was pretty sick at that particular time, but I felt better after I realized what I had done. My nausea wasn't as severe that day.

The slightest bit of interest by other people was almost enough to see me through the next round of therapy. I'd frequently receive more than ten cards and letters a day, many from people at my old high school whom I had forgotten about or didn't even know. Coach Joe Paterno of Penn State and his wife wrote me an encouraging letter, and Frank

Pomarico, the offensive captain of the Notre Dame football team, digressed from the usual Fighting Irish football message to address an article about me in their school paper.

"Notre Dame 44, Navy 7," the article began.

Ara Parseghian, the Notre Dame coach, sent me a personal note, and all the Irish football players autographed the program from the Navy game, advising me to remember the words of Saint Paul: "I have stood firm. I will fight the good fight." All through the 1973 season, I thought that if I was released from the hospital I could still play in the remaining games, and I never recognized it was over for the season until the Army contest was concluded. I thought about football every day, and knowing that the Navy football team and other college ball players still thought about me proved that there was more to life than just hours of dry heaves.

An older, retired officer checked into tower 14 early in December with a surprising diagnosis of massive bone cancer, the doctors finding numerous malignant tumors after a routine operation following an auto accident. He was as new to the whole arena of this disease as I was, and because of the proximity of our rooms, he often overheard my groans in reaction to the therapy. We talked about what we were both going through, and I came to admire him. He was always in reasonable spirits, suffering pain more intense than my own, but no crying sounds ever came from his room. He'd always smile every time we'd get together. He was interested in my progress and knew when I'd be going for radiation and chemo or another test. He told me one day that he admired my perseverance, but there was no way I could thank him adequately for saying that. I was deeply saddened by his death but thankful that I had met a man who showed such appreciation. He was the first person I knew who remained positive and supportive until his death, and this was something I would have never experienced had my plebe year been a regular one.

Commander Jack Renard was the executive assistant to Admiral Mack and a close friend of Commander Smith, and they both talked about how my situation should be presented

Frank Pomerico—Captain's Corner

"Fourth and Long"

Notre Dame 44, Navy 7. Seven down and four to go for an undefeated season. And last Saturday's win was a good win for us because I think the whole school was emotionally down from the USC game.

Well, all that's over and our next challenge is Pitt—and our game with the Panthers might very well be one of our toughest games of the year.

Getting back to the Navy game, though, I've got to say it was great to win. However, after the game I was presented with some very disheartening news about Thomas Jackson Harper, one of the freshman midshipmen.

Tom is from San Bruno, California, just south of San Francisco, and attended the Naval Academy Prep School, which is located in the vicinity of the Naval Academy in Annapolis. In August Tom was a well-built young man, and was the picture of health and happiness.

As a freshman on the Navy football team, he played tight end in each of the plebes' first three games, did a fine job, and showed great potential for the future.

In the fourth week of the season, however, Tom went to the team's trainer, after discovering a lump in his lower abdomen. They took Tom for further tests and found that he had cancer throughout his body and that it seemed to be of the terminal variety.

Well, it's been about two months since his sickness was detected and Tom is still hanging in there, fighting very hard for his life. He is still convinced that he can lick this disease and so far various treatments seem to have cleared up most of the cancer in his lungs. However, Tom still faces an uphill battle. And he still needs a lot of physical and spiritual help.

As I look at Tom's case I can't but think of my own problems and how really small they seem. It seems sometimes that things are not going well—you've just failed an exam, you've had a bad day at practice, you don't feel very good, you've got a cold, maybe you've just had a fight with your girlfriend.

Well, listen pal, look at the whole situation, and ask yourself the question: Is it really all that bad? And the answer is no, it's not.

You still have your health and you still have a chance to come back and do better than you have in the past. So make up with your girlfriend and stick your chin up—because life is as good or as bad as you make it. Of course one will experience setbacks and disappointments, but if we look at Tom Harper's setbacks we see how small our own troubles really are.

I hope we all can look at Tom and see how he is fighting his own setbacks in life—and I hope we can all see his determination not to let this setback defeat him. And in doing this I hope all of us can have brighter and happier outlooks on our own lives.

Looking ahead now to this weekend's game with Pittsburgh— it's going to be a very tough one. We will be playing away from home and they will be out to get us. We've been under pressure before, however, and will show the Panthers what Notre Dame is really like.

So in closing now, I'd just like to say two things. Go Irish, beat Pitt, is one of them. Say a prayer for Tom Harper is the other.

to the Academy. Renard and Smith both thought the superintendent would let me back in and saw to it that my case was not handled in the average way by an impersonal government bureaucracy. Nobody ran to the Navy's Bureau of Personnel and asked what to do. They just monitored my treatment and were flexible enough to think that I might be able to continue with the program. The medical data were an opinion, not fact, and were just one of several recommendations for the superintendent to consider. Commander Renard wasn't surprised that I didn't want to quit the Academy and go back home to California. Perhaps my rationale went back to Plebe Summer, as I identified with the guys who made it through that experience, and the football team. He knew that meant something to me, as if to say, "I've been through Plebe Summer and made the football team. If I'm going to make it, I'll make it here."

Dr. Perlin forwarded a waiver recommendation for six months of limited duty, which I helped him write, to Captain J. C. Hodges, the senior medical officer at the Academy. Some progress had been noted, but there was considerable Navy politics to consider. Captain Hodges knew that as long as I could keep it up, Admiral Mack would do everything possible to keep me. Admiral Mack would have done the same for any midshipman, regardless of affliction, as long as you simply did your best to make it back, one step at a time.

I was very self-conscious about my hair loss and wore a watch cap everyplace outside my room. Everybody recommended that I wear a wig, but somehow the idea of a toupee was uncomfortable—too many cartoons, too many jokes, too many hairpieces lost in a gusty wind.

"A wig? On me?"

"Well, Tommy, a lot of men wear them. You know that. C'mon," Mrs. Hutchinson had replied, and it didn't take long to convince me, especially when most of my hair was gone. A bald head didn't do much for my self-image, and soon a wig and a watch cap became standard parts of my wardrobe.

I was 20 years old on December 12, 1973, marking the event by sleeping fitfully through the early afternoon, recover-

ing from yet another double dosage of radiation and chemotherapy. I had been at Bethesda for three months. I'd
pounded the porcelain sides of my bathroom toilet while on
my knees hundreds of times. I hated chemotherapy. I hated
radiation. I hated the whole cancer procedure. No one had
been definitive about what they were going to do with me,
and the only glimmer of real hope I had was Dr. Perlin's comment that there were some signs, nothing positive yet, but
still a slightly favorable indication that the therapy was having
an effect.

I recognized Dr. Timmons's smiling face from a distance
when I first saw him on the afternoon of my birthday. I was
still groggy from sleeping but was beginning to feel better as
my nausea and the lousy sensations of therapy slowly sub-
sided. It was that lazy time of the afternoon just before the
evening meal. The hallway of the ward was quiet. Timmons
seemed happy, yet I approached him cautiously. What's he
going to tell me now?

"Tom!" he almost shouted. "Admiral Mack called while
you were asleep. We didn't want to wake you, but Tom . . ."
Timmons paused, smiling as he put his right hand firmly on
my shoulder. "Tommy, I've got the best birthday present
you'll ever get!"

CHAPTER EIGHT

Dr. Timmons was always dressed in a Navy uniform, his name etched in blue thread above the breast pocket of the white cloak he usually wore. He reminded me of a product of the eastern prep schools, with young but mature features, dark hair combed with a perfect part, very organized and down to earth. The ward was quiet around us as I looked at him, his smile baiting my anticipation of what he was going to say and putting the sickness crawling through my body temporarily to rest.

"What did you say, Doctor?"

"Tom, today's your birthday, right?"

"Yes."

"I have the best present you'll ever get. You were sound asleep when Admiral Mack called. He told me to tell you that you could come back to the Academy whenever you're ready."

"All right!"

No VA hospital, no doubts about where I was headed, no worries of discharge! I was back to playing football, picking up where I left off in studies, and doing all the things midshipmen do.

Dr. Timmons extended his hand, and I grasped it firmly. "Congratulations, Tom . . . Midshipman Harper."

I thanked him profusely, going back to my room as the daylight of my twentieth birthday gave way to a sunset that cast a clear, soft, reddish glow on the white Bethesda tower.

I spent Thanksgiving Day with Commander Smith and his family over at Coach Tom and Elaine Bresnahan's house just outside the Academy. The table setting reminded me of all the holiday feasts at home, as I gathered with the Smith and Bresnahan clans around a golden turkey. There was a festive spirit in the air, and everyone's mood was too happy to allow any self-pity. The freshly scrubbed faces and eager smiles of the children were a refreshing contrast to the somber stares and routine of Bethesda. I was getting more opportunities to leave the hospital, and love like this was a powerful remedy.

Coach Bresnahan never told me about his first year of coaching at Williams College, when the captain of the football team, a star linebacker for the previous two seasons, literally died in front of his teammates. It had been during the early days of two-platoon football, and one-way defensive players were the stars of several college teams. The Williams linebacker was around his team all the time, to such an extent that Coach Bresnahan felt it was just too much. There are some things you have to face yourself, and after experiencing that player's death, Coach Bresnahan was relieved I didn't have everyday contact with the Navy team. There was no fair comparison to what I had been before the Michigan game. I was a different Tom Harper who said hello now to my teammates, my weight loss, paleness, and wig impossible to conceal.

Coach Gary Tranquil's wife Shirley introduced me to Paula Boyd, an admiral's daughter and a student at Mary Washington College. Paula was one of the original girl cheerleaders at the Academy, and we met after a Navy basketball game. I was almost an old man to Paula, my deterioration bearing a striking resemblance to the regression of her grandfather before he died. She had known him as a healthy, vigorous man, who, once a diagnosis of cancer was made, died shortly thereafter. Paula never said anything about that to me, or about my acne or thinning hair, although cancer had also claimed a high school friend of hers. I had the same physical symptoms. I was still susceptible to increased tumor activity in my lungs and new tumors everywhere else. My liver could rot out, and I'd turn yellow, breathing becoming increasingly difficult as the cancer grew in my chest. I could choke to death. I didn't know why, but I told Paula at a Christmas party that I wondered if I'd be around to see the next one.

She tried to keep me cheery and active, giving me faith in the human spirit and in God. It was impossible to explain why I had cancer and why Richie, her high school friend, 17 years old when he had died, had also been afflicted. Many times during the three to four months we spent together, she would sit patiently and listen, holding my hand as I told her of my goals and dreams. Paula was positive reinforcement and kept negative thoughts away, helping me with building the determination and intent to do what I wanted, and preventing me from closing in on myself, running from any anguish that might lie ahead.

Jack Fellowes was a Navy commander who had reported for duty at the Academy shortly after I entered Bethesda. Sandra Welsh told him about me, and one afternoon he paid a visit to the Smiths' house, where I was spending the day, halfway awake, watching TV.

"Tom!" Commander Smith called as he walked into the room, but I had no desire to move from my comfortable couch and only looked up at them. Jack Fellowes knew it was hard, especially for an athlete, when your body breaks down.

Commander Smith introduced Commander Fellowes as a man who'd just returned from Vietnam after seven years as a prisoner of war. Fellowes had spent months in solitary confinement there. I was sleepy enough that initially what Commander Smith had been telling me didn't sink in. I just remember Commander Fellowes saying as he left, "Tom, it's been my pleasure. Earle, you've got to get this boy out of that hospital. Fix him up with some of these good-looking women around here. He looks pretty good to me!"

I was completely asleep before Commander Fellowes was out of the house. There was a magazine in my lap, with Fellowes's picture on the cover, when I awoke a few hours later, and the ex-POW had written on the front:

> Tom,
> I've heard so much about your courage and spirit. You really are an inspiration to us all. Hang in there, buddy. God bless you.
>   Jack Fellowes
>   CDR, USN

The *Naval Aviation News* devoted 14 pages to Commander Fellowes's story, and I was engrossed in it for more than an hour. He had been blindfolded and beaten and described how the North Vietnamese were masters at rigging the human body with ropes and irons. There was a man the POWs called Straps and Bars, who directed some of the torture, often having another guard jam his foot into Fellowes's back, pressing hard with his leg while pulling on the elbow ropes. One of Commander Fellowes's shoulders was so badly gouged from floor dragging that the open wound drained for three months afterward. Intermingled throughout all of these accounts, however, were a unique sense of humor, trust in God and country, and belief in the positive spirit.

I had met a true American hero with more guts and courage than I had, and he was telling me *I* had courage and determination. I was thinking of the next two years, and here Jack Fellowes had endured seven years of torture, abandoned in a land where people didn't care if you lived or died. His future companionship would be of immeasurable benefit.

Chemotherapy and radiation treatments kept me from going home for Christmas in 1973. Bancroft Hall was deserted and dark then, the hundreds of empty rooms in silent contrast to the happy reunions going on across the country. I was finally able, however, to go home on New Year's Day, to spend 20 days in California.

I carried a football with me, explaining to the stewardess who asked about it that the Navy–Syracuse game had been dedicated to me. We won, and "23–14" was drawn on the side of the ball. I didn't tell her anything about cancer. The pilot managed to flare softly at touchdown, and as he taxied slowly to the ramp I was comforted to be arriving home, but I could not predict how my family would be. What would they make of my wig and wool Navy watch cap?

I was in the middle of all the disembarking passengers, and as I got closer to the door I could sense my parents waiting, sharing anxious stares with my brothers and sisters who were there. They would see a pale figure with hollow eyes and cheeks pocked with remnants of acne blemish, wearing baggy clothes, loose at the elbows and drooping over the shoulders, a stocking cap covering the top of a wig. No one would say anything about my appearance, but I knew I would see it in their eyes. It would be hard to control my own emotions.

I saw my parents first, their expectant gaze changing into smiles and excited waves as Dad leaned over, looking as if he whispered into Mom's ear, "The wig looks pretty good." My sister Sally, a freshman at Cal Poly, Theresa, and Richard were standing next to them, and Jackie, a senior at UCLA, was on the other side, her chin quivering when I looked at her. Everyone surrounded me, hugging me close and shaking my hand.

"How's your protoplasm?" Dad said, in a familiar greeting.

The initial reunion by an airport gate lasted only a few minutes, but it was an ideal remedy for months of discomfort.

Everybody seemed momentarily taken aback by my appearance, and I felt very self-conscious. Jackie started to cry as we walked out of the airport. The uncomfortable aura I had about myself left as I put my arm around her—this was the first time I think I had ever comforted her. Her presence was precious after all the cards she sent and the telephone calls she made, and at this moment she was far more important than my self-image.

Home was a short drive from the airport, the scenery familiar, and the local temperature a special break from the East Coast winter. My older brother, Randy, called from Hawaii, wishing me well after we got to the house, and Mary Beth and my other sister Susie telephoned that afternoon. Denny Follain, an old high school friend, stopped by, and I looked forward to going out to some of our old high school haunts in a couple of days.

I tired easily but wasn't about to think of the chemotherapy and radiation, the nausea and chills. These things waited patiently and inevitably back at Bethesda in the vials of drugs and radiation machines. They were an interruption I would have to deal with later.

We ate dinner that night at the old, long, brown table, the surroundings bringing back memories of when the table was full from one end to the other, eight kids devouring anything that was edible. A big German Shepherd still waited patiently, as usual, under the table, for any scraps.

It was hard to believe what had happened as I lounged around the house and relaxed while looking at old photographs, passing the time in conversation. I had left this house with so much promise, getting ready to start Plebe Summer and collegiate football, and now, six months later, I was back home with cancer.

I circulated with Denny around the Bay Area, meeting old friends and teachers. Everybody knew about my cancer, and I was surprised that many people had thought I was dead. One girl was studying to be a nurse and, more familiar with the terminology than most of my friends, asked questions about the disease and the effects of testicular cancer. She kissed me while we stood in the middle of a fast-food restaurant, and all the other girls with her did likewise, as if to say, "It's OK. We know what you're going through and wish you well."

I went by Oceana High to watch an alumni wrestling match, and later in the day Dad and I drove to Ed Larious's house, where my former high school football coach presented me with a game ball all the Oceana players had signed. Theresa had kept people at Oceana up to date as best she could, putting up with talk that I had either died or lost a leg, and it was with a sense of accomplishment that we drove away, the rumors put to rest.

Time passed all too quickly in California, and after three

short weeks I returned to Bethesda. I didn't feel sad about leaving home. There was no need to look back to what might have been, and my family knew that I had to get back with my recovery program. They had shown their faith in me, especially by not telling me how badly they felt about my new circumstances. Everything they said was about recovery, and I was determined to prove them right.

Earle and Carol Smith lived in a large, three-story, red brick duplex on the Academy's Upsur Road, the small white pillars of the wooden, gray-floored porch greeting passersby. A tree that rose to the second-story windows was set off to the left of the walkway and served as an informal boundary to the other side of the duplex. You could see across the parade field to the Severn River, and the family atmosphere there gave a realistic feel to the Academy business conducted around it.

I spent a lot of time there after coming back from California, usually alternating with the Smiths and the Welshes. It developed into an unspoken thing with everyone—I'd be there without advance notice, walking in to say hello to Carol Smith or Sandra Welsh and their kids. Dr. Perlin had put me on a regular maintenance program, and while there was no place yet for me in Bancroft Hall, Dr. Perlin was willing to release me from everyday residence at the hospital. I'd thought about living with the Smiths or the Welshes, but the idea seemed way out of place. I spent some weekends overnight at Coach Welsh's house, but the layout of the Smiths' home was more suitable, especially with the location of the bathrooms and the way sound would travel. It was uncomfortable to think about getting sick all the time at either place.

Treatment began again, and as usual the nights became longer—chills, the nausea, and a new weakness in my muscles now combining with my thoughts of how to handle the next two years of therapy, while doing everything I had to do at the Academy. It was well past 90 days since I'd entered the hospital, but it was still early in the cycle of drug and radia-

tion treatment. I was uncomfortable at Bethesda, not because
of the care and concern of the attendant staff and physicians,
which was excellent, but because it was a hospital—not the
Academy, not Annapolis or my home town, not a football
field or a library. There had to be some way to manage my
treatment without spending most of my days in tower 14.

Chet Moellar, our All-American safety, brought some
new football recruits to the Smiths' for dinner one February
evening, and I was also invited. Commander Smith and I sat
and talked afterwards. He was particularly helpful to my parents when they had been out, and they thought he was everything a naval officer was supposed to be. Commander Smith
always told them, without being overly possessive or concilia-
tory, "What can we do to help Tommy get better? What can
we do to help him do his work? We'll help him all we can."

I hinted that night about what my status would be, and
Commander Smith caught on immediately, saying, "Hey,
Tom! You can stay here! You can stay with us."

Those were beautiful words to hear, Carol was all for it,
and the Smiths had given me a home.

The Smith kids—Shannon, Jennifer, and Earle Jr.—were
my new little brother and sisters, and only once were they
told of the possibility that my cancer could be fatal. Commander Smith and Carol didn't want to make an issue of the
possibility that I could die in their house, and as far as the
kids were concerned, I was just "really sick." They accepted it
like anything else, and it didn't stop them from playing
around and roughhousing with me. Jennifer, six years old,
was a cute little girl who loved to cuddle up to me. Shannon
and Earle Jr. were a little older and loved horsey rides and
playing around in the yard. They would draw "Peanuts" car-
toon characters on my blue jeans when I fell asleep downstairs after treatment, and it was fun to take them into town
for hamburgers and shakes now and then. I was their own
midshipman, and every little kid on Upshur Road knew it, all
three continually on Commander Smith to get me to remove
my wig for their personal perusal.

They were usually quiet when I was sick, knowing I wasn't the same Tommy who would tell stories or watch TV with them. I spent the rest of the winter and early spring driving the Smiths' little red Volkswagen to and from Bethesda, going by myself until I was too sick to drive anymore. Carol drove me a couple of times, and so did Coach Welsh, who was usually quiet but always seemed to say the right things. We'd talk about football and his Academy experiences but usually shared each other's company in comfortable silence.

I'd first met George Welsh at NAPS. I was with 13 other midshipmen candidates, and we'd been invited to meet the new Navy coach. Most of us had been recruited by somebody else, and we all wondered how he'd react. George Welsh was dressed Penn State style at that first meeting, wearing baggy pants and a mismatched shirt, with striped socks and a funny-looking coat.

We stood in a group, surrounding him while shuffling our feet and wondering just who this man was. He didn't say much, and finally asked Julius Caesar, a talented player from Cleveland, "How much can you bench?"

Julius dutifully answered, and I hid in the background, because even though I had been doing a lot of lifting, I was unfamiliar with just how much I should have been able to do. What if Welsh wasn't impressed?

George Welsh never thought about Tom Harper playing football again because the important thing was trying to help me get well, and he encouraged his staff and all of my teammates to visit. He'd heard the reports like everybody else— three months, six months at best, the spread of the cancer— but he never believed I would die from the disease.

I tried to take an engineering class during the second semester. I'd wear a freshly pressed service dress-blue uniform and drive the Smiths' VW from Upshur Road to the parking lot outside Ward Hall. I couldn't wear my wig, but I made sure I was noticed by the upperclassmen, since the average plebe couldn't drive to class, stroll nonchalantly from the vehicle, and return after class was over to casually drive off. The academic dean had let me take the course, and I studied hard, part of my motivation stemming from his comment that I "should be able to handle it—it's only one course."

I had everything memorized and was holding my own until radiation started again combined with the chemotherapy. My routine had been to sleep in and always arrive late at Bethesda for the therapy, but now I had to go to class first thing in the morning, which made it hard to concentrate. It was almost impossible to study at night, interrupted by throwing up, dry heaves, diarrhea, chills, and nausea. I became self-conscious sitting in the back of the classroom, wisps of hair covering my scalp, and I wore the haunting face of a cancer patient contemplating the next treatment. I felt the stares of everybody and scored a 69 on the four-week exams, one point shy of passing. It wasn't working. Worrying about studies affected my handling of the therapy, so I dropped out of class.

It was a 55-minute trip to the Academy from Bethesda, which was important because reaction to therapy occurred about 50 minutes after treatment. Commander Fellowes told me how the POWs would walk slowly, shuffling their feet, to what they knew was torture, and so I took my time getting to the hospital, driving leisurely and well within the speed limit. Highway 50 was still a pretty journey on the way over, rising and falling so you could see only five or six miles down the road. No billboards were along the highway, and there were several historical markers, the countryside not giving way to development until 20 miles or so away from the Academy.

I never had to wait long for the chemotherapy—Dr. Perlin took care of me. The radiation treatment was often over within an hour, and I'd go straight to chemo, greeting Mrs. Cook, Dr. Perlin's secretary, and then a nurse or corpsman would stick the needle up my arm. There was only one thing to do once the dosage was administered—get back to the Smiths' house and the privacy of my room.

It was a vicious game at times, pushing the Volkswagen well past the speed limit, ever on the lookout for state troopers tracking me from the hidden recesses of an off ramp. I could not wait for red lights nor entertain any driving courtesy, and I stopped only to open the door and vomit some-where along the shoulder of the road. The Smiths' car had no radio, but my intent was totally on speed, music usurped by the obsession to get back to Upshur Road as fast as possible. Any policeman would detect the effects of therapy in my eyes and also the pills in my pocket, and would think perhaps that I was high. I could feel the drugs going into me and smell them all along my return journey, causing a headache and fever, the whiteness of my knuckles visible in the reflection of the windshield. The Academy would find out, and I wouldn't be allowed to drive myself anymore, but I had to drive myself back and forth to Bethesda as long as I could. I didn't like getting sick in front of other people.

I wasn't very sociable after treatment, never saying any-thing to anybody while I went upstairs and closed the door of my third-story room behind me. It was a corner room with a small window overlooking the parade field, from which I watched Vice-President Ford present Navy the commander-in-chief's football trophy for the 1973 season. I stood well be-hind the curtains, throwing up again shortly after watching the ceremony.

I couldn't eat much at the Smiths'. I wasn't hungry, los-ing my appetite after many afternoons and nights of dry heaves. They could hear me all the way downstairs, I was sure of it, as sure as I was that Carol had to clean up the bathroom after me, an ungratifying task, but she never once let on that she found it offensive. Earle and Carol found me at 3:00 A.M. one morning on my hands and knees in the top bathroom, trying to clean up after myself. I was too weak to finish, and they put me to bed, the bathroom fresh and clean in the morning as if nothing had ever happened.

I was still losing weight, and there was no indication that my hair was ever coming back. I tried to eat a bowl of cereal every morning, at times feeling guilty about taking food I didn't pay for. Phil Nelson would visit occasionally, and we took full advantage of the Smiths' VW, Phil hiding in the back seat after a basketball game, driven incognito out of the Yard.

We spent one night drinking beer at a viewpoint of Shirley Highway that overlooks the Academy.

"Phil," I said, "How would you feel if your firstie found out you're up here . . . drinking beer?"

"I'd be scared shitless."

Phil asked me a few minutes later how I felt about having cancer, and I responded the same way, "I'm scared shitless."

Except that if the cancer caught me, who cares anymore?

I did my best to show a happy face, to study, to go to basketball games and have dates, and even to watch spring football practice, standing on the sidelines by myself, sometimes in the rain. I tried to work out, first by walking and then breaking into a slow jog, but I couldn't go 50 yards. I did my own laundry at the Smiths', and it became a struggle to get my clean clothes back up three floors to my room. I had to stop and rest after every flight, and after a while it became a household custom for me to be sitting there breathing hard, my head between my legs as the kids went flying by or Commander Smith and Carol went up and down. They let me do things by myself and didn't interfere with my personal effort, interceding only if it was an absolute necessity. They were respectful of how I wanted to handle it.

Ping pong was a difficult game to play, not because it was hard to direct the ball to its proper place on the table away from one of the kids, but because it was exhausting to have to stand up for so long and move the little paddle back and forth. Carol was painting window transoms one afternoon and I volunteered to help, not knowing the major project she had in mind—painting a little part of the ceiling I would have finished in five minutes had I done it a year earlier. I grasped the brush Carol gave me, climbing the small ladder to make dabs at the ceiling. The brush, laden with paint, was like an anchor in my mind. I tried to press it to the plaster overhead, but it seemed to hang in the air, beads of paint pooling up and dripping down the handle into my hand.

What was happening to me? I could inhale normally but found it difficult to exhale after any exertion. Simple tasks were becoming major efforts. Commander Smith was having serious discussions with Dr. Perlin about my white blood cell count, and both he and Carol had a silent fear about my inability to resist normal disease and the increased susceptibility to pneumonia. I'd looked at myself in the mirror, and their concern seemed to be justified—there were deep, dark circles around my eyes, offset by the pale and yellowish tint of sunken cheeks, my body the very color of the drugs, injected into me. The perspiration on my brow never went away, and if I stood still for too long my body shook with chills, reflecting a man with fever, sickness, and no place to go for a cure.

I went by the Welshes' a couple of times after treatment, and Sandra would leave trash bags for me by the porch door, just in case I didn't make it to the bathroom in time. My diet was still off, and when I went upstairs to the room they kept for me, Sandra would become alarmed—a wheezing sound coming from deep within my throat as I maneuvered up the stairs, my face pale one second and red the next. Was I becoming a burden to these people, the Smiths and the Welshes, getting sick in their homes? Trying to maintain my self-pride, in spite of all the indignities, the throwing up, the deterioration of my body? They didn't seem to think so, but Sandra said in a moment of pity to Carol on one of my more difficult days, "Why doesn't he just die?"

This wasn't insensitive but accurately reflected my situation. Admiral Mack afforded me the opportunity to lean on several fine people. If I could get past the therapy, there was still a hard road ahead—minor, however, compared to the radiation that was discoloring my chest and burning up my lungs, and the chemotherapy that had claimed my hair and sent me to sleep only to wake up sometimes in my own vomit.

I talked about my family with the Smiths and the Welshes, and it helped to get a reassuring phone call or letter from home. I did not want to clue any of them in, however, on what was going on, including Mary Beth, as it served no useful purpose. Commander Smith and I were becoming pretty close, and it was easier for me to say things to him that would have been difficult for my own family to handle. The

Renards would visit often, Commander Jack Renard doing more for me from an administrative standpoint than I could then recognize, his wife Donna assisting Carol in getting me upstairs when I couldn't make it on my own.

While cleaning my room, Carol found Dad's rosary hanging from my bedpost, and I like to believe it made her think of faith in a way she never had before. God was always with me through this episode, I was sure of it, and it would be so good, so comfortable, to say my prayers and be cured. It usually doesn't work that way, and I was learning you had to give of yourself; maybe I was bargaining with God. I told Carol one day that when I recovered I was thinking of becoming a priest. I don't know why I said that, if only in partial thanks for being alive to say it. I'd spent two weeks at a church retreat while in high school, and with the memories of that came the reminder that God made all things possible.

I took the long way to Bethesda once before one of the treatments, heading the opposite way on Highway 495, intent on circling Washington, D.C., to approach the hospital from the other side. It occurred to me, on the approach to the George Washington Parkway bridge over the Potomac, that I could stop the treatment, the therapy, the sickness, and the whole mess by just veering sharply to the right and plunging the red Volkswagen through the railings and down into the deep, murky waters below. It would be simple, and everything would be over. But as I drove closer to the point where I could depart the roadway, I thought it unfair to the Smiths to destroy their car and an unnecessary burden for everyone to come to a funeral—all the midshipmen thinking I'd committed suicide. I thought about all the people I loved—my family, friends—and realized the feelings I would create within them. I don't think it's unusual or wrong for a patient to have brief suicidal tendencies, because these thoughts trigger thoughts of life, of what would be missed if you were gone. You have to decide what is of most value to you, and I tried to give the matter no more thought.

My main goal remained football and the Academy—I

thought about them every day. I lived in a football house, many of my friends were football players, and Commander Smith would tell me, "Those guys are always asking how you are."

It was hard to watch my teammates in practice, since I had been so close, in the best shape of my life, and everybody had said then that I was getting faster and quicker. The starting tight end was tough and an outstanding competitor, but I was 20 pounds heavier and moved larger tackles out of the way during the Oklahoma drills, where he couldn't. He'd had three years on me, but we had both known, and Commander Smith especially, that it was just a matter of time. I would explode at any minute. I remember looking into the mirror, before cancer, saying, "Man, am I ever getting big!"

As the therapy continued, I began to wonder if I'd ever have the opportunity to prove what I could do.

I had a particularly tough week in early spring—double therapy, five days of whole body radiation in the morning, with full dosages of chemotherapy in the afternoon, the mad drive home to throw up and throw up some more, reaching to dry heave. I had to force water down as the perspiration, chills, and lack of appetite were drying me out. The series started on Monday, and by Thursday afternoon I was completely spent.

I hid alone upstairs in my room, staring at a picture on the wall that resembled my favorite Kanaka Creek campsite in California, trying unsuccessfully to keep my mind off the therapy.

I began to think, Man, this is killing me. This chemo and radiation is going to kill me, not the cancer or some disease. I'd heard and now was learning that the cure was worse than the affliction, and this was going to get me. I'd choke to death. I was getting so sick, but nothing would come up.

It was strange and scary to be nervous, dry heave, and shake all together. Maybe the Smiths thought I was faking it, that I wasn't tough enough all alone, a hermit upstairs whose groans and sickness could be heard throughout the house.

This was absurd and comical—everybody was being nice to me, but did they all really believe I'd make it? That I would live? Did anybody care if I played football again? I kept thinking of all the other patients in my old ward at Bethesda—most of them were dead. Was this the way it was supposed to be?

The late-afternoon sun was gone, the darkness of the night bringing a deep emptiness to my heart and developing despair in my mind. I was skinny, flabby, and irritated by all the dry dandruff on my scalp. I felt humiliated at having lost my hair.

I had difficulty breathing, my eyes wide open, listening to every sound in the room. Everybody else in the house was in bed by now, and I could hear the labored effort of my lungs and the increasing rise and fall of my chest. My pulse was fast, and putting my hand over my heart was uncomfortable, my abdomen loosening and tightening with my every movement in bed. I had a different kind of chill, the sheets ice cold, my skin numb. Was I dying? I reached for my rosary, thinking of Dad as I grabbed it, holding it to my heaving chest, my fingers wrapped around the little crucifix and beads.

"Dear God, don't let me die in this house. Hail Mary, full of grace, the Lord is with thee . . ." I continued, and prayed the whole rosary. "Our Father, who art in heaven, hallowed be thy name . . . Dear God!" I'd have to get to the hospital, to the Academy hospital, one half-mile away. They can't find me tomorrow in their house. I did not want to die in their house. I've got to get to the hospital, to the hospital, I told myself. I will not die in this house.

I opened the door as quietly as I could, half holding my breath to hold down any dry heaving, the attempt making it difficult to see, the slight overhead light provided by the heavy, glass-framed opening cut into the roof over the stairs.

I followed the wall down, reaching for it with my hands and descending one step at a time. Was this the way it was when you die—oblivious, panicked, wide-eyed? Had the therapy finally been too much? Whatever it was, the Smiths could not find me in that upstairs bedroom.

I made it to the landing of the second floor, exhausted

and barely able to stand, bracing my back against the wall and sliding down to rest on the hard wood, my fingers numb and my eyelids open but growing heavy. I could make out the scars in my feet, and they seemed to accentuate my bony figure as I slumped to my gut, my head falling forward and carrying me into a blackness where I had never been.

CHAPTER NINE

It was still, outside and all in front of me, down the stairs and throughout the Smith house. There was a comforting presence to the early hour, the silent time before dawn, soothing and assuring me that I was, in fact, quite weak but definitely alive. I rubbed my eyes open, cleaning away the fuzzy feeling by running my hands over my eyelids and the bridge of my nose. My fingers felt thick as I tried to focus on the empty view in front of me, slowly becoming conscious that I was actually staring at the shadows between the stairway and the high ceiling. I must have been unconscious for a couple of hours and stayed where I was for a few more minutes, lying on the wooden second-story landing, my feet dangling over the edge of the next step leading down.

I had the chills, but the nausea was gone, and it was strangely refreshing, shivering, feeling the fresh tingle of goosebumps over my arms and legs. My eyes were accustomed now to what little light there was, and I could make out the way back to the third floor, back to the room I didn't want to be found in. It was quiet, and I was thankful the Smiths were all asleep as I pulled myself up and followed the bannister upstairs. I was tired and aching, but as I crawled back into my soft, fluffy, quilt-covered bed, my thoughts were of deep, comfortable sleep—far away from cancer, death, and the word *victim*.

My alarm woke me at 9:00 A.M., and the Smiths had already dressed, eaten, and left. I called Bethesda before fixing my breakfast, telling the radiologist and Dr. Perlin's secretary

124

that I wasn't coming in for the fifth day of radiation and chemo. I was worn out and not yet over what had happened the night before.

I was no longer able to drive myself to and from Bethesda because I became too sick to drive safely, but it was comforting to sit back and relax and let someone else drive. Al Stanton, assigned to the Academy hospital, was my driver—a big, friendly man with a happy smile and the carriage of an ex-athlete, who'd pick me up at ten in the morning and bring me back to the Smiths in the late afternoon. He was somebody to lean on—always there, saying the right thing with a strong arm to help me when I was too weak to walk. We'd often stop four or five times along the return route, my vomiting and getting sick, I knew, tough and particularly unpleasant for Al to watch.

Al drove several people to Bethesda for treatments; most of the patients elderly and retired, afflicted with heart trouble or arthritis, and diseases complicated by old age. Many of his passengers didn't take many trips. Al kept saying, "Don't give up, don't give up," and asked me, "Do you believe in God?"

"Yes," I responded, a little surprised at his question.

"Keep fighting it. With God, all things are possible. You're gonna make it."

Al worked more than one job to support his family; his children were fortunate, and I saw in him the traits so characteristic of my own father—love of his fellow people and the unbending willingness to help.

"Now listen," I'd say, "you may have to stop four or five times going back today because I'm really sick."

I told him about football, my goals of going back to the Academy and back to playing; it was comfortable to talk with him. He told me he heard his passengers talk so often about how much longer they had to live, be it six months or six weeks, that it was a pleasure to hear something else.

When I finally was allowed to go to the Academy hospital for treatment, I wouldn't need Al to drive me anymore, and I went to see him, saying, "You know what? I can never thank you enough for what you've done. When I get home and out of this, I'm going to write a book, and I want you to be in it."

That one terrible night at the Smiths' did several things for me. It proved I could take the worst of the therapy and still retain enough control of my senses to look out for myself. It proved what determination and the support of other people could do, and, most importantly, it created within my subconscious the emotion that I would live—never mind the side effects or sickness or bouts with depression or how badly I felt. It was impossible not to think about dying from cancer, but it was possible to look past it. I didn't concentrate on dying. Everyone is required to get the most out of his or her life, to contribute something of quality and not to be judged merely by how long they live. I was prepared to die, but I refused to give in to it. There were other things to do, and cancer was not going to deny me the chance to accomplish them. My subconscious mind took control of my destiny the morning I found myself on the stairway landing of the Smiths'. Death, no—dying, no—cancer, maybe—treatment, two years to go. I would do it! Every 28 days for five days—I had to build myself up and get in shape for the next treatment, increasing my resistance by setting goals over the years of therapy, controlling my senses—sight, sound, taste, smell, emotion—combining them into one tool to work for me. Time was on my side, and no matter how bad my condition could get, I would live—never mind the sickening side effects or the disease itself. I prepared to die by preparing to live with determination, dedication, the support of others, and the grace of God.

I was dependent upon the Smiths, the Welshes, and the Academy for so much. I was struck by the irony of it all—to be so reliant on other people, needing them as much as the strength I got from the self-reliant and purposeful upbringing my real family provided. Commander Smith almost carried me to the hospital one night, and one long afternoon I cried out for Carol from the third-story bathroom. I struggled to shower and feared I wouldn't be able to make it back to my room, covering myself with a towel and shouting, "Carol! Carol!"

She raced up the stairs, and I was fumbling with another towel, trying to cover the top of my head as she burst through the door. Carol hadn't seen me without the wig, and she helped me to my room and into bed, never mentioning how bad I looked. She was always there.

The spring of 1974 seemed to last forever, another treatment always around the corner just as I recovered from a previous dosage. The radiation therapy stopped, however, in May. The combination of x rays and drugs had been an experimental one, the radiation costing me endurance and severely reduced lung capacity but perhaps saving my life. Dr. Perlin wasn't even sure. He could recall no one else with such a spread of testicular cancer living long enough to establish any precedent.

I would suffer with the chemotherapy, but without it they said I would die. But would I? I had to trust and believe in someone. We were a team, and by being life-aware I had the defense against the necessary but offensive chemotherapy. It was easy to think about in the comfort of Commander Smith's house, but I'd look at it from a different perspective once I was back in Bancroft Hall. I hoped to be back with the Brigade in the fall and wondered what I'd have to do to catch up with my classmates. Phil Nelson came by often, keeping me in touch with everything; or I'd go get him whenever it was advantageous for him to get away from Bancroft. I wondered sometimes what he would have said to me if I had asked him, "Am I going to die?"

Every time I was with Coach Welsh, I'd be psyched to work out, to push myself and get to the point where I was strong enough to put on pads again. It is hard to put into words just what Coach Welsh did for me. He was the head coach of a major college football team, who, in his first year, took the time, effort, and energy to care for a ball player who had never really played for him and whom he hadn't recruited. Honest and straightforward, he and Sandra took me into their home and made me part of their family, just like the Smiths—my Academy family.

My running fortunately began to improve. I concentrated on putting one foot in front of the other, progressing to a slow jog, resting for 20 minutes after the first time I finally made it around the track next to the eighth wing of Bancroft Hall. The coaches' wives would often stop by if football practice was going on, Elaine Bresnahan, Shirley Tranquil, or Sandra Welsh keeping me company. I concentrated on putting one foot in front of the other, one step at a time, often pretending I was pulling on a rope in front of me, my hands reaching out. Right, pull! Left, pull! Keep going—you have to make it around the field! The next treatment won't hurt as much—build your resistance, Tom! Right, pull! Left, pull! Pick your knees up—try to jog, slowly now—pull, pull! I can see the end of the turf! Pull! Pull! Pull! Right, left, jog, go, go!

I started to jog 50 yards, walk 100, jog 50, walk 100, and finally at the end of spring I made it around the whole circumference—440 yards. That was not very far for a football player, not actually very far for anyone, but a goal had been achieved, and I set another as I finished—to make it around four times without stopping. It took two months, but I did it before leaving for the West Coast for the summer.

The Naval Hospital at Oakland was advised of my condition, and along with my medical record I carried a letter of introduction from Dr. Perlin about my case history and his request for the type and frequency of dosage. I didn't need my wig and watch cap this time, since my hair was slowly growing back, dark and curly. I looked forward to going home, grateful for the unique circumstances that had allowed me to live with the Smiths. I was one of them, not an untouchable, but just "sometimes sick" to the kids, and their constant activity and youthful exuberance had been undeniably therapeutic.

My family had not seen me react to the therapy. I hadn't received any chemo during my last visit and tried to explain how it would be. I couldn't have them waiting on me as if I

was a tired, sick, old man. Dad drove me for my first treatment, and I promptly introduced him by opening the car door
and throwing up on the asphalt of the Oakland out-patient
parking lot.

"It's tough," he said, in a calm and sensitive voice, not
needing to say anymore.

The best trips were with Denny Follain, my old high
school friend, and Denny and his van were a welcome part of
that summer. He knew what to expect, and we'd have a leisurely drive over, listening to his stereo and talking about old
times. He'd have the motor running when I was through with
the treatment, the door open for me, radio blasting as he'd
race the machine out of Oakland. He'd turn down the radio
volume when I started to feel badly, the van's padded uphol-
stery soothing and comfortable as we sped home. He'd wait
to call me a couple of days after the therapy and was always
ready with a friendly and uplifting comment. He'd seem to
know when I felt better. Denny was like Phil Nelson in that
way, and although I never told them both directly that I
needed them, I'm sure they knew.

There wasn't a weight room available at home during the
summer, but I started an aggressive running program, and
my body quickly advised me if I was working out beyond its
limit. One morning I woke up super-psyched and ran to the
public park down the street to do 45 minutes of calisthenics,
followed by running and running and more running—or at
least so I thought. I must have stopped and lain down to rest.
I can't remember when or how, because I woke up in the late
afternoon, the bright sun gone and dusk settling in. I was
more exhausted than anything else, but it surprised and
scared me to have unconsciousness come so quickly.

The left side of my chest started to hurt badly, exactly
where there had been a concentration of radiation. I had to
get back to Bethesda. I couldn't lift my arm to comb my hair.
Was it some sort of serious relapse? Another tumor? I'd have
to get it checked out by Oakland first, but how much did they
know? I didn't want to go through the whole story with them.
I needed Bethesda but didn't want to worry anybody in my

family, and I had planned on attending Denny Follain's wedding. It was important, for all Denny had done with the drives and his companionship, but more importantly, cancer was not going to interfere with my schedule. I resolved to put up with an Oakland Naval Hospital review and head east after the wedding.

I did my best to clue people at Oakland in on my situation, but their examination was inconclusive and unfriendly. "Possible relapse," they wrote in my medical jacket, recommending immediate followup by Bethesda for further examination of tumor recurrence throughout my left chest wall. It was unnerving news, cold and impersonal, and I had to sit through another lecture by the radiologist there, who wondered whether or not I knew just how serious the situation was. I knew what he was talking about, I'd heard it all before, but the pain made me believe what the Oakland people had to say. They were ready to admit me immediately into their hospital, but I promised to head directly for Bethesda after Denny's wedding.

I didn't have to wait to see Dr. Perlin since I had called ahead and scheduled an appointment on a nonclinical day, and, as usual, he was right on top of the situation. Dr. Perlin was a good man and a good friend, very busy with his research, teaching, and daily clinical duties. He made me feel as if he had no other patients. I don't know where he got all the time to do all that he did.

"Midshipman Harper's here," Mrs. Cook would tell him, and he'd greet me with a handshake, a smile, and 1000 folders on his desk, always asking how I was feeling and how my running and workouts were coming.

Dr. Perlin listened to my description of the pain in my upper chest as I sat in his office, and though he was concerned about my complaint, there was marked improvement from the last time I'd seen him. I'd regained some weight and sported something of a tan, a pleasing contrast to the whiteness of his examination room and the paleness of my skin from months before. I wasn't wearing the wig and sported a nice moustache.

The familiar surroundings of Bethesda told me I was back home in capable hands; Oakland had been too cold, too impersonal, and I was just another body for them. I trusted the people here. They would identify the source of this new pain. Dr. Perlin referred me to a pulmonary specialist after his initial examination, and I was introduced to Dr. Dorstella Travis.

The pain had worried me all the way back to Bethesda. Sitting there in front of Dr. Travis, I kept thinking, Oh, no, not more chemotherapy, more drugs again—please, God, no. What if they had to start radiation again? The doctor was very professional and courteous, and appeared genuinely concerned.

"Well, Tom, how are you doing?" she asked, smiling.

"Sometimes I can't raise my arm," I replied, shrugging my left shoulder.

She studied me for what seemed to be a long time, not saying too much.

"Do you think there is anything wrong, Doctor?"

"Let me take some x rays, first," she said, and as I prepared for them I wasn't sure what was happening. I was scared, and there was little, if anything, I could do about the situation. I kept thinking about that awful radiation chamber.

Shortly thereafter, after a quick but careful check, she gave me good news—the pain was caused by radiation scars, a buildup of inert tissue. I had accumulated a mass of tissue because of all the radiation administered earlier, the heavy dosages burning my lungs to the extent that my breathing capacity would never be the same again. All that worry, about a relapse or another tumor or maybe even the collapse of some vital organ, seemed silly now, since her diagnosis was made fairly quickly. The pain began to fade, and I learned that it's always better to have something checked out than to endure the mental anguish indefinitely.

Soon afterwards, I tried to be more friendly and cooperative in the treatment process, even though I was thinking, I've got to go through this again?

There were patients who didn't follow a regular program, harming themselves, but I'd only missed one appointment.

There was no way I could know more than a physician with years of formal training and even more years of actual practice. I'd talk with some patients who'd go into how they'd begun to question the credentials of doctor after doctor after doctor, because of something they'd heard or read about. I didn't like hearing other patients talk about how many doctors they had been to, and I was especially thankful that Dr. Perlin and I had developed mutual trust.

I wasn't about to be a victim in a fight where emotions and trust are often deciding factors, regardless of age, background, or stature. Death wouldn't make me a loser to the disease, and I resolved to approach things completely out of my control by doing my best, as if I would live forever, but living every day as if it were my last.

I had been away from the Academy for almost three months. It was late August of 1974, the hottest and muggiest time of the year for Annapolis, and the new class of 1978 was receiving the full treatment as Plebe Summer drew to a close. The varsity football team was in the middle of its second practice of the day when I came back to the Yard, and Sandra Welsh and Carol Smith were in the stands watching practice. I took a seat a couple of rows in front of them, but initially they didn't recognize me. It had been more than a year since my first Plebe Summer had begun, and by all rights I should have been out on the field as the starting tight end and an upperclassman.

Several people had not expected to see me again. But I was back, my spirit refreshed as I watched practice; and I felt, after everything that had gone on, that I couldn't have been better prepared to put aside the idle days of summertime and take on the challenge laid out by Admiral Mack. It was time to go back to Bancroft Hall.

I was glad to see everybody, and although some of my teammates seemed hesitant at first to talk to me, I didn't mind. It was a natural reaction, since I was supposed to be dead.

I knew it was time when Captain Forbes, the commandant, also watching that afternoon's practice, commented to

Carol about the length of my hair, telling her that the Academy couldn't let up on me once the academic year started. I wanted to stay with my class—1977—but it would be difficult. Perhaps they would let me wear third class shoulder boards, even though I'd be going through plebe academics once again. I'd missed eight full months of school and didn't look forward to a full year of plebeian chores—quite a contrast from offering comfort to a dying admiral at Bethesda and daily rapport with medical officers.

My new classmates were talking about things I'd already done. I'd had my Plebe Summer, and while at Bethesda and living with the Smiths was encumbered by all the rituals of that fourth class year. It hurt to see Phil Nelson wearing third class shoulder boards because, as far as the Academy was concerned, I was still a plebe. They assigned me to a new company, and though I requested to be situated in the first or second wing of Bancroft Hall, closer to the academic buildings, my new company, the 17th, was located in the seventh wing, as far away as you could get. I was introduced to the new plebes as a turnback, who'd had to miss plebe year because of "personal problems," and I certainly didn't look as big as my teammates and the upperclassmen had remembered me.

It took a couple of days for me to move back into Bancroft Hall, and both Sandra and Carol were there to help. It was hard moving all my gear, my lungs aching with the exertion, and I wondered how I was going to handle the rigors of fourth class year if merely moving my belongings was hard work. Sandra Welsh thought it was a strange sight; who at the Academy had ever heard of the wife of the head football coach actually helping a 20-year-old plebe, who wheezed, huffed, and puffed like an old man, haul his belongings into an elevator and up to his room?

Dr. Eichelberger, still the team physician, turned my treatment over to Bruce Ruppenthal after talking with Dr. Perlin. Dr. Ruppenthal was familiar with my case and had been assigned to the Naval Academy after completing three years of internal medical residency at Penn. He had gone full circle, from a small Quaker school in college to the military atmosphere of USNA, and he spent most of his time at the Academy hospital, whether it was with a mid magnifying a minor illness to get out of exams or with a serious problem involving severe illness, a medical board, diabetes—or cancer.

He was a cheerful, professional physician, of average height and build, with a special sense of humor, a lovely wife named Letty, and the type of person who, right off, instilled in me a concern about getting better rather than getting worse. I liked him and Letty immediately, and he coaxed me into becoming a bargainer, a productive negotiator with my treatment, to maintain my individuality and humanity, not becoming another number for the case file of embryonal cell carcinoma.

I had to schedule treatments around plebe year, so not only were the five days of actual therapy an interruption, but also the two weeks it took to recover from the chemotherapy. Another series of treatment would begin just as my body would be returning to normal. I didn't want a master–slave relationship, and so I had to put myself on equal footing with the doctor. Otherwise, I could not handle the requirements of plebe year—the academics, the discipline, the come-arounds and events, the rigid schedule, and physical standards. If I didn't handle the chemotherapy correctly, I would let down Admiral Mack and all those who had helped me get back into the Academy. I remembered the problems I had just taking one academic course while living with the Smiths, and I didn't want to fail again.

Despite the cancer and regardless of the Academy's generosity, it was still difficult to accept being a plebe. I'd already been through something far more demanding than rote memorization and knowing my place at the lowest point in the chain of command. I would be 21 years old soon, and when my older brother was my age, he'd been a first class. I had enough to worry about with the chemo and studies to waste time with the new problems of 17- and 18-year-olds. I never accepted this new plebe year, but it was the price I had to pay to realize my goals. I told myself I'd do anything to beat cancer, and when I thought about that, the disgust I had with fourth class year paled in comparison. I would absorb the discipline I didn't need, if only to acquiesce to the early rules Admiral Mack, in essence, was laying out.

I asked no special favors before beginning things all over, and other than allowances for my treatment, I wouldn't have expected the Academy to give me any. I was expected to perform as any other member of the class of 1978, and I had to create the image that all I was concerned with was academics and plebe duties. It was a delicate balance, as many of my new classmates didn't know what my situation was, and I didn't want to tell them where I went every month.

I didn't want to talk about my cancer or dwell too long on the subject, because in the back of my mind I would recognize it only as the word—*cancer*—nothing right or wrong about it. My subconscious didn't know I was trying to be positive about it. It just knew I was emphasizing *cancer*, and I didn't want to be that type of patient. My doctors would do everything possible to influence positively the course of my treatment, but the ultimate conclusion of the whole process was up to me, the patient. I was worth saving; I figured I deserved to be living; I emphasized life, not death, and tried to replace fear with enthusiasm; I set goals and had a purpose, not the least of which was to get back on the football team and prove Admiral Mack right by successfully completing the curriculum. I was intent to go about my business and do what was important to *me*. I had to feel good about myself, because my thoughts and thus my response to the outside world were dependent so much on my emotions. Good thoughts were good health, and it didn't seem possible that there was such a thing as talking positively about my cancer, as my mind only heard it was a concern. I would gain absolutely nothing by thinking about *cancer* all the time. I had to be receptive to getting better, and the chemotherapy was easier to endure when I was in a proper frame of mind.

Trying to play the plebe game and keep my head above water with the academics, therapy, and the effects of cancer upon my body, combined with my agonizingly slow workouts, made me appear aloof to my fellow plebes, my new classmates, and I was at times a stranger to the team spirit fourth class year instills. I had a choice and didn't have to apologize for my ego, and I didn't want anybody to feel sorry for me. I concentrated on how to react and was more interested in results than in methods. Life and death are future events, and I thought about what I wanted to happen—playing football, graduating, becoming a naval officer. I didn't need the few people who were well intentioned but were always offering pity to patients, continually looking for people to feel sorry for. I felt better with people who responded to challenge and wanted to help others back to fulfilling the purpose in their lives, and it was for this reason that I did my best to be a regular member of the brigade of midshipmen. I'd wake up at night during the therapy periods, sick, knowing I'd be doing the same thing the next day. I had to talk to myself, keep psyching myself up, mix persistence with therapy, recovery, and the daily pressures of plebe year.

My first squad leader had been on the football team with me the year before but now was no longer playing because of a knee injury. I was happy to hear he would be the first class closest to me and went to his room, entering with, "Hey, what's happening?"

"Now, Tom," he responded, looking at me hesitantly and a little surprised, "I know you were on the football team, and so was I, but . . . you've got to treat me like every upperclassman. You've got to have a plebe year . . . and don't call me by my first name. You know how a first class is to be addressed by a plebe."

I stood there, staring at him. "Hey, what?"

"That will be all, Midshipman Harper."

He turned his head away, a signal for me to leave, which I did, without saying "Sir," without saying anything. He went to see our company officer after I left, telling him he couldn't have me in his squad since it wasn't fair to either of us.

I hadn't anticipated this reception and was directed to another squad at the next formation. After the muster, I found myself looking down at a short first class, his hat pulled over his eyes and seeming, from the way I was looking at him, to rest on his nose.

"Mr. Harper?"

"Yes, Sir?"

"I'm your new squad leader. Do you know who I am?"

"You're Mr. Twelpin, Sir."

"Come around to my room after dinner."

"Yes, Sir."

This guy wasn't too friendly. I felt uneasy eating at his table, and to make matters worse, he was my own age. I asked myself why I was going through all of this again and massaged my pride as I knocked on his door to fulfill my come-around. Midshipman First Class John Twelpin graciously let me enter and stood up, all five-foot six of him walking over to stand in front of me.

"Mr. Harper, you have been specifically placed in my squad, and you are my special assignment."

CHAPTER TEN

The statue of a proud Indian has looked for half a century upon the off-white, brick courtyard to the front of Bancroft Hall, the bronzed face a silent sentinel of the midshipmen walking past. It rests upon a tall marble base, and Tecumseh, as it is called, is painted with water-based colors before premier athletic and social events. Tradition guaranteed that academic fortune was bestowed upon those thoughtful mids who tossed pennies at the statue. It was, however, not so much for the classroom assistance that I looked to Tecumseh, but more for the milestone it served to be on the way back to my room and the plebe tasks prescribed by Midshipman First Class John Twelpin.

I wouldn't return to the class of 1977, and while some firsties held back, a few upperclassmen were determined to see that I had a full plebe year. One former classmate who accompanied me through my first plebe summer wouldn't even shake my hand, lest he "spoon" me (the handshake symbolic of the dropping of class distinction, and common at the end of plebe year). My company officer anticipated my aggravation and was an easy man to talk with, but he also felt I needed fourth class exposure for the next nine to ten months.

We were told the purpose of the plebe year was to cross the gap between civilian life and life as a midshipman, "to instill discipline . . . develop leadership qualities, and . . . introduce nautical, aeronautical, and military aspects of a naval career." This purpose was significant and impressive to young plebes, but not something a plebe quoted when asked about such a different college life style.

Plebes were awake before 0500 (5:00 A.M.), busy with uniforms, room cleanliness, and memorizing rates before the 0600 formation in the hall. The third class duty section marched us down to breakfast, which was quickly consumed, in relative peace, before the 0705 come-around. We performed that perfunctory task for ten minutes, the closing of such duty accentuated by the first early chow call, that quick recitation of meals, movies, officers on duty, and upcoming calendar highlights for the upperclassmen. I ventured, psyched for the chore, into the hall, with the task of informing everyone in our corridor, booming out in a clear voice, "Sir! You now have ten minutes until morning formation! The uniform for formation is working uniform blue alpha! Formation is outside! The menu for noon meal is ginger pot roast, pot roast gravy, buttered egg noodles, broccoli spears, lettuce, cucumber, tomato salad, French and Italian dressing, whole wheat bread, coconut cream pie, iced tea with lemon wedges! The officers of the watch are: the officer of the watch is LCDR Donley, 10TH Company Officer! The assistant officer of the watch is LCDR Stephenson, 23RD Company Officer! The midshipman officer of the watch is Midshipman First Class Gallagher, 6TH Company Commander! The battalion officer of the watch is Midshipman First Class Houlihan, 18TH Company Commander! The movies in town are: at the Playhouse, *Bananas!* At the Plaza, *The Stewardesses!* At the Circle, *Jaws!* There are 88 days until Navy beats the hell out of Army, 109 days until Christmas leave, 264 days until the second class ring dance, and 268 days until first class graduation! Sir!"

I repeated the same things at the five-minute call, abbreviated it slightly at four and two minutes, and finished the one minute, rushed version, after reminding everyone, "Turn off all lights, running water, electrical appliances! Lock all windows and close all doors!" yelling to a feverish finale, "Time, tide, and formation wait for no man! I am now shoving off, Sir!!!"

I had four morning classes—English, sea power, chemistry, and navigation, the final period spent on the upper deck of Griffith Hall, a location that couldn't have been worse for a plebe. Griffith Hall was the academic building farthest away from my room, and there were only 15 minutes from the ring of the class ending bell until the noon come-around routine. The navigation professor would lecture straight to the end, leaving no extra time to roll up your charts or disassemble and bag your equipment, and it was at least a quarter-mile to Bancroft where, once inside the doors, we sprinted down the corridors, squaring each corner with a resounding "Beat Army!" All this was getting rather old.

I changed as fast as I could into my "grease" uniform, an exact replica of what I'd worn to class but a uniform set reserved only for certain formations and inspections. We were always sweaty, and it never failed that an officer of the watch had changed or the menu was wrong, interrupting a carefully memorized litany. My roommates and I gave each other the proper shirt tuck, brushing off lint and any other residue before we went out the door to our come-around, giving our chow call, having our inspection, and finally marching to the mess hall. Plebes served the first class and kept up the supply of food to the table as long as possible, holding up trays or pitchers for more food or tea; lunch and dinner were served family-style. Plebes were, of course, the last to eat, and if there was any ice cream, a fourth classman could forget it.

"Mr. Harper," Twelpin said, early in the year. "Why are you on T-tables?"

"Sir, I'm on the football team."

Twelpin acidly digested my remarks, replying, "No, you're not. You don't practice with them. You don't play any games. Why do you need to be on the T-tables?"

I didn't say anything as he continued, "You don't. Starting this evening, report to my table and sit next to me—every meal from now on. If you have any objections, I'll take it all the way to the Commandant."

"Yes, Sir."

Twelpin was taking away an important ingredient of my recovery program. T-tables were training tables for the sport in season, and plebes eating there didn't have to worry about how they ate or how they sat, avoiding the rigid, sit-on-the-edge position of their not-so-fortunate classmates. Most importantly, there was plenty of food for everyone. My weight was starting to come back, and now I had to sit with Twelpin.

He was right. I did not suit up for or play in any football games, and although I could complain to one of the team captains, I didn't. They had enough to worry about, and I reported to Twelpin's table, answering his questions and serving everyone, but eating only a little of my own meal. I asked permission to leave, and Twelpin was slightly surprised.

"Mr. Harper, aren't you hungry this evening?"

"Not to eat here, Sir."

"Very well. I can't force you to stay. By the way, what are the movies in town?"

I told him and left, going to the T-tables where my friend Steve Scott had saved me a plate. It became a pattern—eating little with that wimp Twelpin, excusing myself, and then heading for the T-tables where my friends were.

There were two academic periods after noon meal, followed by intramurals or varsity sports until the evening ritual of come-arounds, chow call, and formation. I warmed up during practices with the team during football season, and when they broke up for separate drills I began my program. One day I would walk and run around the turf, and on other days I would alternate with 5-, 10-, and 40-yard sprints. Commander Fellowes would often be there, and we talked about a lot of different things. He told me about some of the tortures—the wire around his wrists and feet, being beaten for hours while tied to a chair set three feet off the ground, crashing repeatedly to the deck. He learned, as did many of his fellow POWs, to absorb the blows and roll with the punches, but there was nothing to absorb when the side of his face or the back of his skull hit the hard concrete floor. Commander Fellowes could touch hands with his arms stretched straight out behind his back, level with his shoulders, courtesy of the North Vietnamese. I felt comfortable telling him about my own struggles and was inspired to try and run an extra lap after talking with him.

Academics was a key ingredient not only for my education but also as the cornerstone for staying in school. Without passing grades, I wouldn't graduate, receive a commission, or remain a midshipman—regardless of cancer, the therapy, or the many people who gave their support. Midshipmen have a substantial course load—mathematics, chemistry, physics, seapower, the professional sciences, English, to name a few— and plebe indoctrination was woven throughout the academic schedule, not allowing much free time. If a plebe could antici- pate questions or assigned tasks, the load was lightened, but there was not any foresight that could protect against vindic- tiveness or immature use of authority. My grades, however, surprised more than a few people, including me.

John Twelpin was conscientious but was more concerned with doing things according to strict regulation than with practical or common sense. My return to the Brigade seemed a mistake to Twelpin; I was not physically qualified and should not have been readmitted. It was that attitude combined with a "little man" complex which made me dislike him; there was never any of the fear and respect typical of so many plebe–first class relationships. Twelpin was an annoyance, serving as part of the difficulty of reaching my goals and reaf- firming the legitimacy of Admiral Mack's decision.

"What are the parameters of the sparrow missile, Mr. Harper?" I'd find out and tell Twelpin.

"What are the characteristics of the Polaris class sub- marines as compared to the new Trident class?" I'd find out and tell him.

Front-page articles, back-page articles, sports-page arti- cles—I gave my daily report, but instead of showing any real interest in the content of what I had to say, John Twelpin was more interested in putting me through a drill as his subser- vient reader.

"You will have a plebe year," he kept saying to me, aware of the fact that I'd miss half a month of Bancroft routine because of the therapy, thereby easing out, to him, of the re- quirements of fourth class life. He thought he was my "father figure." It was some comparison.

Most of my uniforms had to be retailored because of my weight loss, and I was still wearing the loose-fitting summer whiteworks when the Brigade switched to blues. This was a sore point with Twelpin, and he picked up on it about the time a heat rash developed on my right thigh and along the lower side of my back. He was after me in particular to wear the service dress-blue uniform for evening meals and grew increasingly irritated when I kept telling him that my blue uniforms were being "recut."

He'd say every day, "I want you in the proper uniform, Mr. Harper. What is this?" Perhaps it bothered him that I stood out in the squad, a fourth class in white, off-balance with the dark blue attire of everyone else.

I put toilet paper under my clothes to cover the rash, keeping it from moving through to the surface, as I was bleeding from the irritation. My roommates, Buck Wickland and Andy Cuca, would help me undress during come-arounds, peeling off my trousers with fresh paper ready, my skin rough, ugly in places, with little bubbles and pockets that oozed a clear fluid and a yellowish substance along with the blood. I had the shingles—herpes zoster—aggravated by the chemotherapy, as painful a hurt as I had ever experienced, and now I had to juggle that along with the chemotherapy, hospital routine, nausea, sickness, academics, and my plebe rates.

My lack of a proper uniform started to wear thin with some of the other upperclassmen in the company, adding fuel to Twelpin's interest, and when my clothes finally arrived from the tailor shop—clean, reshaped and freshly pressed—I gingerly pulled the virgin material of my trouser leg over the tissue and freshly carved skin. The shingles were ugly, and running sores were on the flank of my thigh, slivers of pain shooting up and down the middle of my back. My tie, shirt, blouse, spit-shined shoes, and cap went together well, and I proceeded to visit Midshipman First Class John Twelpin.

"Mr. Harper! You look great! So professional!" he said, scrutinizing me from head to toe. I wanted to reach down and grab his tiny throat.

"Just fine, Mr. Harper, just fine. Don't you feel better?" I didn't smile as I looked into his eyes, my face expressionless while the insides of my wool pants rubbed my thighs raw.

"Yes, Sir. I feel great."

I went back to my room, each step feeling like my legs were being pushed across broken glass. Andy Cuca helped me into a chair, my face ashen white and palms covered by the sweat from the outside of my fists. I undid my belt buckle, and Andy pulled at the bottom of the trousers as I eased out of the top. There were pieces of bloody skin on the inside of the seat, as if somebody had spilled raspberries all over the inside of my pants and stepped on them.

"My God," Andy said, but I finally had the upper hand on Twelpin. He no longer seemed a threat to me, and anything he tried to do was a reflection of his own problems. I was readmitted into the ward that night.

I attended class on days two and four of the five-day regime of chemotherapy, but it was very hard to concentrate. I walked from the ward, past Hospital Point and over the green wooden bridge toward the academic complex, stopping along the river crossover to rest. There were places plebes weren't supposed to walk or sit, but if it was the shortest path to my destination or the nearest place to rest, I usurped the privilege, too sick to answer and too tired to move or explain whenever confronted by an upperclassman or an officer. When I rested between Sampson and Michelson Halls, classmates would occasionally ask, "Hey, Harper, waiting for the gouge?"—the term symbolic of inside knowledge of what the next test might cover. It was the same way in the Bancroft elevators, off-limits to midshipmen except first class in the late afternoon. Many days I was not able to make it up the split concrete stairs of the seventh wing and had to use the elevator, generating a look of surprise from an officer or a firstie who happened to be an accompanying passenger. The excuse for my presence was guaranteed by a permission chit that stated, "Permission to use elevators due to chemotherapy."

I scored an 85 on the first chemistry exam of the semester, the grade circled in red at the top right-hand corner of the first page, but to this day I don't remember taking the test. I recognized the handwriting, the style with which I'd done the calculations, and even the ink of the pen I'd used to sign my name. How could I have forgotten the hour it took to take it, much less the time involved in study? I frequently reviewed material after "lights out" with a flashlight under the covers or beneath the cubbyhole of my desk, sometimes even behind the curtain in the shower. Did I forget all of that? I never went to class again during the days drugs were sucked into my arm.

Doctor Ruppenthal was very frank and honest when we first met. "You've still got a long way to go, Tom," he said, aware that the statistical chances of recovery were less than 8 percent. He was never negative, even with unfavorable news, and he reiterated that the chance the disease would prove fatal was an opinion, not fact, and that he couldn't forecast his own death, much less mine. He made sure, unknown to me, that well-qualified nurses or corpsmen were present before, during, and after treatment, and he was never late to any of our appointments, setting up therapy around my Academy schedule. If I wanted to wait so I wouldn't be sick during a football game, we moved the treatment one way or other, even to a Saturday or Sunday night, no matter what time it was. The waiting for treatment wasn't easy, both at Bethesda and at the Academy hospital, but simply knowing that Dr. Ruppenthal was busy and would get to me as soon as he could really helped. Ruppenthal set up one routine for 10:30 A.M. Sunday mornings at the hospital, right after church, but he was on vacation for one session, and his substitute didn't show until 3:30 that afternoon. The only thing his replacement said was, "I slept late."

This turned me off so much that the treatment was one of my worst; maybe I was spoiled by Dr. Ruppenthal, but this other physician just gave me the medicine and left—no human contact, no apology, sloughing off my concern. He may have been a busy man, but he wasn't worth much as a physician by treating his patients merely as the object of his mechanical skill.

Head Nurse Darlene Webster was a stickler for detail, not in a harsh way, but I couldn't seem to get through to her. She wouldn't allow any food in the ward other than during normal feeding hours. I couldn't use the ward kitchen, and

Webster would wake me up during regular meal hours, telling me to eat and that if I didn't there wouldn't be anything until the next meal. But I couldn't eat since I was either throwing up or trying to be perfectly still so as not to be miserable. Sandra Welsh, Carol Smith, and Donna Renard kept me steadily supplied, however, with "illegal" snacks, and I had Dr. Ruppenthal to thank for getting my diet back to an acceptable level. The Academy hospital staff didn't have much experience dealing with cancer patients in the midshipmen's ward, so it was rare when I could eat three regular meals a day while undergoing chemotherapy. Every four hours I was awakened for temperature, pulse, and blood pressure, but Dr. Ruppenthal talked the staff into ignoring these vital signs whenever I was asleep. He also secured access for me to the small kitchenette on the floor, so I could scrounge real food behind Webster's back.

I surprised Nurse Chris Picchi, who had been transferred to the Academy hospital from Bethesda. I spotted her on the hospital staff roster, where it indicated she was working in intensive care. I'd wanted to talk to her ever since that first night in the Bethesda recovery room, and when I said hello, she was very startled to see me. She explained a few days later that she thought I was dead.

My roommate and I were studying for a midterm chemistry test late one night, and just before taps I reached into my desk drawer and took out a couple of pills.

"What's that?"

"Codeine."

"Are you sure you really need them, Tom?"

"Hey, Andy, the last few days I've been taking them right before bed, and I've slept well . . . great dreams, and I wake up without a bad thought on my mind."

Andy looked at me curiously. Did he think I was getting hooked on these things?

"No way. I just took them for shingles," I replied, before he could say anything more. I wasn't dependent upon those pills, even though Andy thought I was. A couple of days later I reached into my desk drawer and came up empty—I was out of pills. I asked Dr. Ruppenthal for some more, but he couldn't believe I'd gone through the whole bottle so fast. It was the day before my scheduled monthly drug treatment, and he told me to wait. That night I wasn't able to sleep and spent the hours with hot and cold flashes all over my body. My eyes didn't want to close. I couldn't relax, and I felt as if a bag of sugar had been injected into my veins. Andy was right; perhaps I was addicted to the codeine. I collapsed in our room the next day, right before noon meal; the lack of codeine and that morning's chemotherapy were just too much. Andy hurriedly brought Twelpin and our company officer to my side, and they called for a corpsman, lifting me onto a stretcher and carrying me to an ambulance; Twelpin even looked concerned.

Dr. Ruppenthal weaned me slowly from codeine during the next few treatments. I'd started taking the drug to ease the pain of the shingles, and withdrawal from it took place right as I was getting sick from the chemotherapy. I didn't want to get hooked on the codeine forever, though, and chose to endure the pain.

Admiral Mack was pointing me, as he did with all midshipmen, in the direction of truly knowing a sense of duty, but more importantly he was helping me in goal orientation, as my preoccupation with the challenges of plebe year kept my subconscious from emphasizing cancer. When told I couldn't do what I wanted to do because of the therapy, I took it as a personal criticism, putting me on the offensive, to fight and regain lost ground.

I worked with Dr. Perlin and Dr. Ruppenthal on the response to the Medical Board inquiries, the input going through the Academy staff and on to Washington. Although they could have discharged me at any time, or kept me in the Navy until therapy was completed before discharge, Admiral Mack sold them on the idea of letting me stay. As long as I kept up they would retain me, sufficient enough reason to approach the tasks of fourth class year without dwelling on the fact that I'd been through some of it once before. The Medical Board at the Academy took their time responding to the paperwork, often taking six months to a year to respond. I couldn't have received better cooperation from the leadership at USNA because they didn't let the medical opinion tell them what to do.

Little things helped me realize that plebe year wasn't going to last forever. Commander Smith helped with the reports about my condition, and most everybody I talked with was supportive and wished me well. Delores Faulkner, who handled my medical records, greeted me with a beautiful smile and words of encouragement whenever I needed my file. Captain Coppidge, the athletic director, had seen to it that the Naval Academy Athletic Association picked up the tab for my parents' stay at the Bethesda lodge. Every now and then, while I was in the hospital for treatment, the association would send over a basket of fruit. Sandra Welsh agonized over the Medical Boards, and she and Carol Smith came to see me in the hospital more than anyone else. They knew the days to visit, when I would be feeling good, and when I was in no condition to see anybody.

I told all my profs at the beginning of the year that I would be missing from seven to ten days of class each month. I didn't want them to feel sorry for me, but at the same time I needed to let them know in case I was late with homework or missed a gouge session. My company officer informed most of them about my situation, so it was no problem arranging for extra instruction or taking an exam in an off hour. James Abbot, my mathematics prof, was especially appreciative of my protocol, even though I usually completed his assignments a week late. Prof Abbot had a friend who was an admiral and a top man at Bethesda who, by regulation, had to recommend me for physical discharge. But he was also quick to point out to the Academy and Bureau of Medicine that they did not have to accept such a recommendation. I wasn't aware I deserved such treatment.

I don't believe any of the profs "gave" me a course. I took seapower under Lieutenant Commander Gordie Peterson, and we were a month into the semester before I asked to be excused due to the therapy. Profs like Peterson were good listeners and went along with my requests, just like the hospital

did with my setup of the therapy. I still had to meet the
course load and post acceptable grades, while my profs rear-
ranged their own schedules and adjusted their own deadlines.
I occasionally studied for exams over at the Smiths' or
Welshes', and little Kit Renard even took it upon herself to
read to me from my seapower book. I wasn't able to keep
most of the same professors during the second semester, and
rather than go through my explanations one more time, I just
became known as the mid who was always gone.

I went to football practice as often as possible, working
out daily around the practice facilities. I was put in charge of
the Navy football mascot. I was the goatkeeper, along with
another ex-football player, of Bill, the honor voted on by the
team and coaches, usually going to a player who had used up
his eligibility or had been injured and could no longer play.
Bill provided sufficient incentive for me to keep up with the
workouts. I had to be strong enough to run with the goat
from under the goalposts to the middle of the field and over
to the sidelines. Since the Army–Navy game was on national
television, I didn't want to embarrass myself, Navy, and Bill
by collapsing in the middle of the playing field before the
game started.

Life in Bancroft Hall was a structured, regimented exis-
tence, but it was left to each individual midshipman to suc-
ceed or fail. The Yard was a self-sustaining community. Once
a week I dropped a mesh bag full of dirty laundry out into the
hall, and it magically reappeared, fresh and clean, a few days
later, although at times the cleaners appeared to have been
chewing on my clothes. More than 4000 mids ate three meals
a day at the same time under the same roof, the caloric intake
such that if you weren't careful you'd end up on the weight
control program. Every event was scheduled and publicized
with exact timing, from parades to bus traffic for away football
games, from holiday meals to pep rallies, from class registration to end-of-semester exams. There wasn't time to tag along
for a free ride through school. A mid had to prepare for a term
paper, chemistry and math tests, tough swimming classes, a
mile run for time, and professional requirements such as uni-

forms for formation and signal flag tests—just a few exam-
ples—and often all in the same day.

Since the cancer had spread to my lungs, it could just as
easily spread, once in the blood system, to any other part of
my body. I'd had numerous bone scans at Bethesda and a
brain scan with good results, but the liver and spleen scan still
showed tumor activity. There was some decrease in the size of
the tumors in my lungs as radiotherapy was stopped, and by
the middle of plebe year any major advance of the disease had
so far been held in check.

Dr. Dale Rank, a physician I would meet later in Texas,
had a meaningful explanation. "Tom," he said, "cancer is as
natural as the sun rising. It is woven into the fabric of what
we are and is not something mysterious that comes out of the
dark. Cancer has evolved as a product of life and reproduc-
tion. The normal rejection of cancer cells is automatic—white
blood cells and/or antibodies usually attack and destroy the
cancer cell. Antibodies can reject the cancer cell, or they can
protect it. Blocking antibodies are required for pregnancies
and bone marrow transplants, and what they do with cancer
is not something bad but something misused. Everything has
its equal and opposing force, and positive emotion has a salu-
tary effect, perhaps causing a chemical reaction, as has been
proven to occur with negative emotion."

What Dr. Rank was telling me was not a fairy tale, that
cancer was a simple affliction and could be cured by a positive
attitude. A patient should not be in deadly fear of cancer. It is
of immeasurable benefit to understand and play an active
role, as a partner, in therapy. Positive emotion helps everyone—even those who die as cancer patients. An unnecessary
burden is placed on both the patient and the doctor by passive
fear. There are more things a patient can be told if he or she
takes an active role. It should never be a role reversal, where
an antagonistic relationship between doctor and patient su-
persedes a partnership or cooperative effort. Cancer is never
easy, and Dr. Rank and most of the medical people close to
me helped smooth my fears by carefully stripping away igno-
rance of the disease.

I was the only male midshipman in recent memory to have a positive pregnancy test, which excited Dr. Ruppenthal, not because of a sensational medical find but because the test would serve as an excellent tumor marker—a tool he could use to track the progress of the chemotherapy. Cancer tumors generated an abnormal hormone normally produced by placenta tissue, which normally wasn't found in a urine or blood sample unless the patient was pregnant. Whenever there was any doubt about how I was doing, they would get another HCG level. The closer to zero it got, the better the indication.

My white blood cell count was another sort of tumor marker, in addition to measuring my reaction to therapy and susceptibility to infection. They also tracked HGB, hemoglobin, the oxygen-carrying ability of the blood, trying to determine by means of a centrifuge test the number of red blood cells in my body. Dr. Ruppenthal was concerned more about having too little than too many. My platelet count had to remain high; it was my defense against bleeding, the platelets forming the meshwork on which a blood clot forms. Spontaneous bleeding obviously would not help me in any way. Dr. Ruppenthal did other tests, looking for any protein in a urine sample (a sign of kidney damage), looking for sugar in the same sample (a sign of diabetes), looking for ketones (a breakdown product of fatty acids that indicates the body doesn't have enough glucose to burn adequately, causing the body tissue to break down fats to get the sugar available; it was typical of starvation).

They did many other chemical scans, all of them serving to assist in measuring my progress. Exploratory surgery was a popular technique at the time, but once Bethesda saw the extent of the spread there had never been a need to open me up. The disease was above my diaphragm, and in cancer ranking I was stage III, not very good. The chemotherapy continued in an experimental procedure for which I had to sign a release.

I can still feel the tightness of the rubber tourniquet around my upper arm and the coldness of the alcohol as Dr. Ruppenthal or one of the nurses cleaned off the vein in my forearm before the insertion of the needle. It was hooked up

to the IV bottle, and very slowly, a little at a time, contents of
the syringe tied into the line were injected into my body.
There was little pain in the application, only the sickness that
followed, and I learned how to handle it better as the treatments progressed, by lying down, staying still, and not moving around. Every now and then I'd get out of bed, easing out
through trial and error, and I didn't go through the violent
inner upheavals of my body. I would vomit, but gradually,
and then it was back to sleep. Or I would just lie there, not
saying a word as the hours went by. The only good result of
my Oakland visits was viscerile, an antinausea drug. I didn't
want any extra needles stuck into my body, and at first I refused to take it, but viscerile certainly worked. I exercised as
hard as I could before chemotherapy, pumping myself up,
bringing tone back to my upper chest and arms, and a few
times the viscerile needles broke off in my arm; my muscle
was too tight to allow penetration. I used the drug in modera-
tion, the viscerile helping me sleep, and researched as best I
could the quadruple combination of new drugs that now com-
prised the chemotherapy—velban, dactinomycin, chloram-
bucel, and methotrexate. What I found out didn't scare me
but provided a better understanding of the whole process.

Charlie Tongue was the field equipment manager for the
football team and was assigned the daily responsibility of taking care of the Navy mascot. Charlie was a 30-year veteran of
the Academy, a short, heavy, jovial man with close-cropped
hair and a twinkle in his eye. He was an accomplished handy-
man, driving an old pickup loaded with odds and ends and
yard paraphernalia, and he would do anything for you, spar-
ing the time from his home and beloved garden to help anybody out. Charlie was a cancer patient, but nobody knew too
much about his treatment because he was quiet, always smiling, and in good spirits. He was a living example of positive
emotion and just before his death, when he was given a game
ball by Coach Welsh, in a poignant locker room meeting with
the football team I realized that the Naval Academy will always stand for something good.
        I worked out hard for the Army–Navy game by running

and lifting weights. The weight I could push was nowhere near what I'd done at NAPS, and the effort hurt, but it was worth it when I thought about what I had to do. I met President Ford at the game and managed to steer Bill through the Army formation. When another midshipman, Bill, and I led the Navy team onto the field, my lungs felt as if they would burst. My last breathing tests had shown I was moving less than 50 percent of the air I should have been able to inhale and exhale.

I was definitely stronger, however, than the year before, savoring every faster step and every extra pound of iron I could lift. I was working out one cold night during the Dark Ages, the time between return from Christmas leave and spring break. An ex-NAPS teammate asked if I was disappointed that the weight training I'd done at the prep school was all for naught. I was skinny, still down almost 30 pounds from my playing weight of 225, and I started to respond that, yes, it was hard, that I never dreamed during those long exercises that I'd be like this less than two years later. But I remembered all the comments from Bethesda about how my physical condition was a major factor in my staying alive.

"No," I responded, "not really."

I often walked alone around the Yard that winter, around Farragut Field or on the Astroturf, waking up at 3:00 or 4:00 A.M., slipping on a pair of sweats and quietly leaving the company area by the back stairwell. Sometimes I would act out a touchdown or a great reception while cursing my predicament. Why me? Why in God's name was I going through all of this? Why was I picked? What a goddamn waste! I still couldn't believe it and prayed it was all one bad dream. I'd watch the waves of the Bay, the white caps beating themselves against the rocks, breaking the silence of the dark. I sat on a rock and thought about working out, or a professor, or chemo, wondering what it would be like once the treatments were over. I dreamed of suiting up again, actually putting on the helmet, the shoulder pads, slipping thigh pads and knee pads into my pants, making sure my socks fit just right. I dreamed of that first day back on the field—catching passes with Steve Scott or blocking Julius Caesar, helping George Welsh build Navy a winner, and repaying him for helping me out. Then there was plebe year, and I thought about how the stress really doesn't matter when it comes to life and death, and that being a fourth classman was just another game to be played.

I'd written Dad earlier in the year to explain that I'd done my best but that being a plebe again was ridiculous. I knew the system and the whys and wherefores of its methods, but I was ready to leave Annapolis because virtually every day it seemed I was repeating things I'd already done. There was no need to answer to people my own age. If I'd wanted to do something at NAPS I did it, but it wasn't that way at the Academy. Something would finally go right, however, making me feel better, and I understood later that there was something meaningful to Admiral Mack's intent. I never mailed the letter.

I thought about Twelpin. How would he be as an officer? Would somebody throw him overboard or shoot him in the back? I would think and think and think, and afterwards run back to Bancroft Hall, feeling good and ready—ready for a test, ready for chemo, sneaking back up the stairs, back into my room, and under the covers.

I continued to lift hard and increased the intensity of my workouts up until the last minute before leaving for the hospital, since that way I could rest during the therapy and measure my progress from treatment to treatment. I'd compare how much I'd lifted from one chemo period to the next, confiding in Dr. Ruppenthal about my personal goals and desire to play football again. He was like a brother to me, never once saying anything discouraging about what I wanted to do, quiet for a few seconds, then broadening into that sly grin of his to say, "You know, Tommy, you'll never know if you don't try."

Bruce Ruppenthal took care of me in subtle ways, from detailed conversations with Dr. Perlin to the positive inputs he always gave the Medical Boards. He wasn't a career Navy physician, but he volunteered to serve, absorbing the military with a wry wit and gaining the respect of his patients for his true concern. He invited me into his home, and he, Letty, and their kids were as much family to me as the Smiths and Welshes.

I made progress with running and soon could jog slowly all around the Yard, sometimes alone but more often with friends. There is tradition throughout the Yard, and at every turn there is a monument to some past glory, echoing the courage of lives given in service. This was more than motivation for me—it was a lesson in appreciation for what I had—my life. So many others never had the chance to mature and plan for the future, enjoying life for what it really is. I was building myself up and the chemo would tear me down, but there was always the opportunity to be better than before, to come back, and it was a constant battle between my body and the drugs. I was walking back from the library with Phil Nelson one afternoon and felt extremely weak as we approached the first flight of stairs. I was scared that I couldn't make it up one flight to the first landing. I wanted to stop, but Phil said, "Goddamn it, Tom. This is bullshit. You're going to beat this. C'mon, Tommy, you're a football player."

I had to do something, and we walked up together.

Besides football, Bancroft Hall, academics, chemotherapy, and everything else, I met another Navy nurse. I was taking the March treatment, checking in at the nurses' office, when I first saw this beautiful, blond Navy lieutenant. I thought I knew everyone on the hospital staff, but I had never seen her before, and Dr. Ruppenthal came in while I was writing down the usual information on my check-in sheet. I acknowledged her to him by moving my eyes in her direction and nodding my head toward her side, and he answered my quizzical gestures by raising his eyebrows a couple of times and flashing his patented grin, telling me later that she was Jewish, single, and living with a dentist.

I tried to impress her with my knowledge of Judaism during the week she was assigned to me.

"Du bist shain," I said to her one evening, which caught her attention, but she replied something I didn't understand. My day-old knowledge was rather limited.

Our conversation by the end of the week, however, developed to where I thought she might say yes if I asked her out. She had a couple of days off after her last day on the day shift. I timed my exit from an adjoining restroom as she left the nurses' station, extending my hand and saying, "We should get together sometime, outside this hospital."

"I'd like to, but I'm living with somebody."

"I know."

"I really don't think it's possible, Tom," she replied, and left for the weekend. But on the last day of this particular treatment, Jacquelyn Burgin left a get-well card on my bed, enclosing her personal card inside with her telephone number written on the back. My last treatment that day wasn't bad at all.

A fourth classman can't date regularly. There are specific weekends, definite time periods, distance limits, and a curfew. We were allowed, though, to bring dates to the Masquerader's Theater in the Yard, with a 0100 sign-in. Jacquelyn and I went to one play, but we left before the conclusion of the first act and drove to Georgetown for dinner. I was out of limits and out of uniform, but it was worth it.

We began to see more and more of each other, Jacquelyn becoming my friend and counselor. She decided to leave her dentist friend and rented an apartment just outside an Academy gate. The very personal and special times we spent together helped with the chemotherapy, inspired me to lift and get ready for football, and built my confidence. I had lost a testicle, part of what distinguished me was gone, amputated by a surgeon's scalpel because it was engorged by a malignant tumor. Testicular cancer asked me questions. Am I still a full man? Am I masculine? Can I perform? Will I ever get married? Why can't I be like all my friends, have a good time, and not have to worry about whether a girl is going to think less of me because I only have one testicle?

I could identify with women who had mastectomies, but I was a football player, a midshipman, a young "macho" man expected to perform. Breast removal was more publicized and in the media, out in the open; women were telling all, and many organizations would help any woman who asked. It

was embarrassing to talk about losing my testicle, and I sometimes felt ashamed, but Jacquelyn was my confidante, and I
asked her what she thought.

"Jacquelyn, does it bug you . . . I mean, do you think any
less of me because I have . . . well, you know, only one testicle?"

I was embarrassed to ask, but her frankness really made a
difference. "I don't even think about it, to tell you the truth,
Tommy."

I sighed in relief, and Jacquelyn picked that up immediately. "You know, Tommy, you can have sex. Yes, you can
be a father. Don't worry about it. Hey, look at it this way.
People may find out about you. With testicular cancer out in
the open, more men might become aware earlier that they
have it. I know that doesn't help you right now, but if they
found out early enough they wouldn't have to go through
what . . . you know . . ."

"What I have to do?"

"Yes. You keep talking about life and contributions and
all. This could be your contribution."

Jacquelyn and I spent our best hours after she'd worked
the late-afternoon shift. I'd sneak out of my room at night,
and we'd walk along the Bay seawall, holding hands, sometimes not saying a word, and other times I'd talk about all the
plebe hassles, telling her story after story.

I was secured from a number of plebe rates during April,
not having to run down the middle of the halls or square corners anymore, with no more chow calls or come-arounds, and
even Twelpin left me alone. I was studying hard, working out
as best I could, trying to play off fatigue from the late hours
and therapy while in class. Jacquelyn was somebody I needed
to be with, and we spent many hours together during the
spring of 1975. I'd sneak out of the Academy between classes
and visit her apartment.

We were sitting by Trident Light along the rock seawall in
the dusk of an early evening, when a first classman appeared
from across Farragut Field to inquire why I, a plebe, was out
there in the first place, with a girl. Lieutenant Burgin turned

around, the silver bars on her uniform catching the firstie's eyes, as she said, "Please leave us alone."

"Yes, Ma'am," he replied, and walked gamely away, startled at the evaporation of his command presence. I had to smile at him.

Often on Friday or Saturday nights, when I supposedly was studying in the library or undergoing extra instruction with a prof, I enjoyed a gourmet, candlelight dinner at Jacquelyn's small apartment. We'd laugh about Twelpin and what he'd do if he found out, or make fun of some of the other upperclassmen. If they only knew!

"Well, Jacquelyn, you know if Twelpin found this out he'd have a fit. I can see him now, sitting in his room, in his underwear. He's probably shining his shoes and thinking about what I can do for him."

I was walking a fine line as far as the regulations went, but this was an interlude in both of our lives, and I took no moral claim or stand as we shared nothing but great times together. Dr. Ruppenthal was casually aware of our relationship, but he knew that Jacquelyn was concerned about my chances of living and what cancer could do to us. It was a delicate matter, and he counseled her in a tactful and sincere way, advising her not to get too emotionally involved. There were no guarantees he could give her, and I certainly had no intention of causing Jacquelyn any hurt or concern.

The chemotherapy and my reaction to it were becoming as routine as the three daily formations, taps, and the infamous pop quiz. I looked forward to Youngster Cruise, at sea onboard a fleet ship stationed off the West Coast, and since I was cleared for duty, the summer training would fit in nicely between treatments. Commanders Smith and Renard had me psyched to go, relating some of their mid cruise experiences full of hard work, humor, and learning the real Navy beyond Mother B. Plebe year closed on a note of satisfaction, and I had accomplished one goal. I was no longer a fourth classman. I had contended with cancer treatment and the plebe routine at the same time and had not asked any favors. I didn't consider myself any tougher for it, knowing that repeating the year was a price to pay toward recovery. I didn't need the discipline or the harassment, especially Twelpin's kind, but there really was no other way. I joined a group of fellow third classmen en route to the USS *Higby*, a destroyer homeported out of Long Beach, California.

When I first saw the *Higby*, she listed to port, the faded gray paint of her bow peeling and split, floating in water coated with an oily substance, and I noticed rust-like residue all along the water line as we walked up a creaking aluminum and wood walkway to her quarterdeck. The vessel sailed for San Diego in the morning, yet it didn't appear she could make it out of the Long Beach harbor.

Our quarters were stacked four feet deep and two rows wide, and as there was limited room in the small lockers, I didn't bother to open my sea bag. It was hot below decks, the summer sun baking the topside and steadily sending its heat down the ladders to reflect off the bulkheads. There was something wrong with that ship. The crew was desperately trying to fix her old engines, and the noise was incessant at night, scattered red lights in the passageways emitting beams that coated the humid air, adding a dismal glow at knee level to everything I could see. If I sat up in bed I'd hit the person above me, and if I moved to the right my face pressed against the bulkhead. Two of the crew jumped ship in Seattle after they'd put their fists through her hull.

I had nightmares at night, waking up in a hot sweat, and looking for a way out. I was up for learning as much as I could about the fleet, but not this way. I didn't mind work, sweat, or duty, and I spent two days cleaning out gun turrets with a sailor called Wolfman, the best member of the crew. The *Higby* wasn't working for me, and I'd resolved not to waste effort with the things that didn't work toward my recovery. It was hard to get around her creaking hulk, and though I could jog around the Yard, climbing up and down ladders and meandering throughout passageways took a lot out of me. Going to and from the ship was a major effort, and it took me almost five minutes to walk up the gangplank.

I flew to San Francisco on the first three-day weekend,

and when I arrived home I knew I wasn't going back to the *Higby*. I checked into sick quarters at nearby Moffet Field, dizzy, the noise of the *Higby* ringing in my ears, her peculiar smells surrounding my body. I didn't care if the *Higby* reported me AWOL, I didn't care what the Academy thought; that ship wasn't helping me at all.

I called Dr. Ruppenthal, who knew where I was. He'd already processed paperwork for the West Coast hospitals if I needed it. "Tom?"

"Doc, you've gotta help me. I'm not going back on that ship. It sucks. The noise is driving me crazy, and I can't stand it. The only reason I'll set foot on it again is to get my clothes. I'll be back for treatment July 9."

CHAPTER ELEVEN

It was a two-and-a-half-hour drive to the Stanislaus River, its tree-lined banks and cold, fast-moving water a perfect haven from the USS *Higby*. Denny Follain called after I'd been home for a few days, his idea of a raft trip undeniably refreshing compared to the disillusionment of my abortive Youngster Cruise. The *Higby* had been a bitter letdown, her incessant noise ringing throughout my dreams as I slept in my parents' house. Navy life had to offer something better than that vessel, regardless of whatever effect cancer therapy had on my compatibility for sea duty. First Class Cruise, two years away, would give me another opportunity.

The winding gravel road down to the river reminded us of the movie *Deliverance*, Denny and I brushing off a local gas station owner's inquiry about our experience and equipment after we'd asked about the best entry point. There were three girls with us—Denny's wife, Diane, his sister, and a friend from high school—and they would meet us a few miles downriver, after we started our journey from an upriver path that led down to the water. Denny parked his van on the wood and concrete-tiered bridge crossing over the southern river entrance, and the girls waited for us to pass by while we carried the raft some 200 yards down a steep dirt embankment.

The water was incredibly clear, and as I caught my breath while admiring the beauty of the river, Denny asked, "Tom, are you sure you're ready for this?"

"I'm ready, Denny."

I was psyched to make this trip, but right at the start we began to have trouble.

There was a fork in the river before the bridge, and we tried to navigate our way to the right to get back into the main stream, the current deceptively fast next to the shoreline, as we belatedly realized when we couldn't steer ourselves in the right direction. Our rubber raft circled downriver, our laughter and exhilaration with the splashing, chilly water sprays changing to uneasy concern as the raft headed directly for an outcropping of rocks, trees, and brush on the other side of the bridge. We had not recognized this from the road above, and the rocks that had appeared so slippery wet and inviting combined now with rush of the river to tip the small raft oars out of our hands. Denny and I could do nothing to stop it.

The river pushed us past three large boulders, the first stopping us, the second spinning us around, and the third lifting the raft upside-down. I was exhausted before reaching the surface but thanked God for the buoyancy of the raft, holding on to the side rope as we were flipped into the air, the raft offering a helpful boost as I struggled to the top. Denny was OK, rising up almost simultaneously, and we tried to hold on to the raft, grasping for brush to avoid being swept downriver.

We were in a bad position, pinned between the raft and fallen trees that just nudged the surface, trying to hold the side ropes with one hand and the tree limbs with the other. The raft was moving fast, back and forth, hitting us in the face, and we let it go, helping each other to the treetops as Denny kept asking if I was OK. I wondered how we were going to get safely back to shore, because the nearest bank was 60 feet away and the rushing water and slick rocks made it a dangerous journey. Denny would have to help me cross. I was too weak and knew immediately I'd exceeded my endurance. I had almost no strength left.

Diane thought at first we were playing a trick on them when they saw the raft go by, that Denny and I were crouched low, hiding from their view into the raft. We weren't in it, and as they looked upstream they saw us being thrashed by the fast-moving water as we struggled to hold on to fallen trees and brush. It would have been fun—riding downstream with the current—had I never had cancer therapy, but now it was up to Denny to get us out.

The girls reached the river bank and waded out as far as they could into the river, stopping on the rocks at the current's edge. I could see them moving frantically around, yelling something as Denny came hand-over-hand along a smooth tree side toward me. We decided that he would go first and find the right rocks to walk on.

I followed Denny along a log, both of us treading sideways to the strong current. I was totally dependent on Denny, and he pulled me along. Denny didn't stop and I was able to follow his momentum out of the water and onto the rocks. It was slow moving, since I had to rest after every other step, and we cautiously walked the distance to where the girls were standing, placing our feet ever so carefully on the wet stones. I was feeling better as we edged closer to safety, but I knew I didn't have anything left if we fell back into the river. We managed to get to the bank, and Denny and I both collapsed. I realized I could have easily drowned, and from that point on I never forgot my limitations.

Dr. Ruppenthal had my new orders processed, which directed me to report back to the Academy. The *Higby* was notified that I wasn't coming back, but I did stop by briefly to pick up the clothes I'd left onboard while she was dockside in San Diego. I was greeted by the watch officer when I reached the quarterdeck.

"I thought you were supposed to be a big Navy football player," he said sarcastically.

"I'm here to pick up my clothes, Sir," I replied, leaving topside and going below decks for my sea bag. I didn't look back as I left that ship. Commanders Smith and Renard had talked so often about how great their cruises had been, and I wanted that experience, but right then it just didn't happen for me.

Jacquelyn was worried, my letters telling of dismay about my first introduction to the fleet, as my doctors questioned my physical stamina and condition. I had a high temperature during the last few days of my visit home, and I carried the fever back to Annapolis. I wasn't feeling well when I checked into the hospital, but Dr. Ruppenthal diagnosed the infirmity as strep throat. It was always that way with cancer patients— even ordinary illness caused everybody to worry.

I had chemotherapy, of course, during July and August, but when I wasn't in the hospital I organized my schedule to spend as much time as possible with Jacquelyn. I devoted many hours to lifting weights, and she would give me rub-downs at night after I'd worked out most of the day. I was sore, both from the exercise and the lingering effects of the chemo, and I relaxed in Jacquelyn's apartment. Jacquelyn lis-tened, cared for my concerns, and shared with me the thoughts that affected my confidence—thoughts of playing football, handling the therapy, and combining that treatment with the increased difficulty of upcoming third class year aca-demics.

I was working out in the eighth wing weight room one late afternoon, a building thunderstorm casting shadows through the overhead windows and onto the barbell equip-ment lined against the wall. A cooling wind accompanied the gathering clouds, the drop in temperature coming just as foot-ball player Ray Crevier and I finished a hard set together. I was through lifting for the day, and the change of weather created a reflective mood as I rested on a small bench pad. The football team was back, getting ready for the two-a-days of summer practice, and I had been working out with them as much as I could. I wasn't able to compete in any of the drills or to keep up, but I was in considerably better shape than the year before. It had been a good summer, notwithstanding the abortive cruise and my near drowning.

"Ray, do you think I'm a fool trying to play again?"

"I'd do the same thing you're doing now, Tom. You've gotta fight."

I was late for practice one morning, having spent the night with Jacquelyn, and many of the football players teased me about it during practice. I realized there had to be a change in my priorities. Jacquelyn was becoming a threat, not in an intentional, harmful way, but a threat to my goals of playing football, graduating, and receiving my degree and commission. I couldn't pinpoint the reason exactly. Maybe she wanted a deeper relationship, and we talked and talked, but we were missing something. It was nice to have her companionship and share our lives together, but my original priorities were being hurt, and that was something I could not afford. We agreed to see other people once in a while, and my trips to see her became less frequent. I started dating other girls and went almost a year before seeing her again.

Admiral Mack retired in August of that summer. He would have done anything in my behalf, even lobbying Congress if BuMed pressed for my discharge, and he wanted the new superintendent, Rear Admiral Kinnard McKee, to be as supportive of my efforts as he had been.

Admiral McKee was a fair, inquisitive person with a penchant for knowing how things were run from the bottom up. He met with several members of the Academy staff, military and civilian, concerning my status, concentrating on my medical progress and academic standing. My records were favorable, and while some of the testimony was mixed, Commanders Smith and Renard were of the most help. They had discussed many ways of handling the new superintendent, and they were present at the meeting Admiral McKee convened before the start of academics where a decision had to be made. Was I to stay there, or was I not fit for duty? I'd seen the new admiral watching the football team practice, unaware of what he'd heard about me. Everybody I knew told me not to worry about what could happen when Admiral Mack retired, but I didn't know Admiral McKee. What if he was an officer who went strictly by regulation? Or if he felt I belonged at some other place, at home, or in a VA hospital?

"Admiral," Commander Smith said, "the only thing that's keeping that boy alive, outside of his own courage and determination, is this school. Without it, it would be not very good, I'm afraid to say. This school . . . this institution, the Academy, gentlemen, is what's keeping this young man alive."

Admiral McKee looked at everyone in the meeting, the

grouping of senior officers in summer white uniforms accentuated by the dark green felt covering of the table around which they all sat. He paused briefly, then leaned back in his chair, saying, "Well, as far as I'm concerned, Tommy Harper can stay here until he either dies or graduates."

I became closer to Dr. Ruppenthal and his family during third class year. He and Letty lived in housing provided by the Navy across the Severn River from the Academy, and one of my proudest moments was the day I ran from Hospital Point up past the hospital and other staff housing, through the main gate, out of the Academy, and down over the drawbridge leading to Highway 2, turning right on the other side of the Severn River and onto the road that led to the Ruppenthals' house. The run was a little more than seven miles and very slow, but it was the longest run I'd made in more than two years.

I was more than a patient to the Ruppenthals, more than just a friendly midshipman who happened to have cancer. There was that special something that existed with the Smiths and Welshes. I was a part of their family, with a love, concern, and closeness as real as my true parents, brothers, and sisters. What a special chemistry to have combined with these families just at this time and place!

Dr. Ruppenthal and I went fishing a lot, and once went with a corpsman in a small boat powered by an even smaller outboard motor to test our luck in the waters of the Chesapeake Bay. We didn't catch anything, but time passed quickly as we traded sea stories and off-color jokes. We laughed about a previous excursion in the Severn, when we were almost swamped trying to get out of the way of a larger craft down by the drawbridge. We agreed that we owed our survival then not to luck but to our expert seamanship.

That expertise, however, didn't prevent us from getting into near disastrous trouble again. The winds were calm throughout most of the day, picking up ever so slightly in the afternoon, much to the delight of several sailboats that had been virtually dead in the water. But clear sky gave way to overcast, and when the first sprinkles of rain hit us, we knew a severe nautical error had been made. The three of us were in a small rowboat with limited power, within sight of land but almost in the middle of the Chesapeake Bay, our vessel riding low in the water because of our overgross combined weight and provisions of cold beer and sandwiches. We had checked everything before our expedition except the weather forecast.

The sailboats all around us began to pick up speed, and Dr. Ruppenthal put our motor to maximum throttle, pointing our 16-foot craft toward shore while we held fast, our little bow rising and falling with a steady whomp-whomp sound as we skimmed across white caps, heavy rain chasing us from behind. Our sailing companions were falling right and left, the colorful sails of the smaller boats hitting the water like an open barn door on a windy day. We started to take on water ourselves, and I grew concerned about how far it was to land. Dr. Ruppenthal's hair was matted to his face, the rain mixing with the spray of the Bay to drench us thoroughly. "Half a mile to go, boys!" he shouted, grinning through the storm as the little engine behind him worked itself past redline.

The Stanislaus River was fresh in my mind as our boat finally ran into the dock, Dr. Rupp closing the throttle just before impact. We left the soggy food behind, and shouting goodbye through the blowing rain to our corpsman, made a direct line to the comfort of the Ruppenthal house.

I barely had time to dry off when I was asked to babysit. Letty had scratched her eye with the point of a hot comb while tending their little girl's hair. Dr. Ruppenthal took her to the Academy hospital for treatment of the cornea abrasion, and I took care of the kids, fixing tacos for everybody. There was still plenty of food left over by the time they returned. I'd put the kids to bed, and Letty retired early, so Dr. Ruppenthal and I finished off the remaining tacos and talked. Football, my progress with running and lifting weights, what Dr. Ruppenthal wanted to do once he completed his Navy tour, cars, women—we talked about a little of everything.

"Do you think I can really play football again, Doc?"

"Yes, why not? Your endurance isn't what it used to be, but so what? I think you should give it a shot."

"Can I have kids?"

"Well, your other testicle was shielded during radiation, and there hasn't been any cancer activity with it. But who's to say, Tom? You should get a sperm count, and I think it would probably be favorable."

"Would my kids be OK? I mean . . . if I ever got married, would my wife and . . . you know, children . . . would they be normal?"

"They'd be all right, Tom. Your cancer cells couldn't live in my body any more than mine could live in yours. Their chances for getting cancer are like mine, and, well, everybody else's. Who's to know?"

We talked about attitude and life style, reaction to things outside your control, goals, emotion, doing the things you wanted to do. He nodded in agreement as I told him about my own plans, the chemotherapy, and especially the routine at Bethesda. There was only so much one man could do, and I told Dr. Ruppenthal I believed God was watching over me.

"Yes, Tom, I believe he is," he replied, smiling. "He has given you the determination of three men."

We transgressed into other subjects, Dr. Ruppenthal mentioning that my therapy was progressing well and that they'd be taking a serious look at stopping the chemotherapy soon. I went to sleep that night in an upbeat, positive mood, noticing my watch indicated 5:00 A.M. when I turned off the light.

Youngster year is an in-between year. A mid is too old to be subservient, too junior to exercise direct control, but at least I wore a new shoulder stripe and had put the frustrations and hassles of plebe life behind me. I couldn't escape the academics, and didn't really want to, but studies became a second priority as my treatment progressed through the fall of 1975. Coach Welsh pulled off a major upset as Navy beat highly ranked Penn State, and I passed the season again as the goatkeeper. I worked out harder and was pushing 200 pounds, the heaviest I'd been in two years. Physics, engineering, lab work—I was doing below-average work, but I managed to cram in enough extra instruction to come out favorably at term's end. I reversed myself the last two years of school and carried better grades in most of my courses. Youngster year, however, my goal was not grades but to get back into good enough shape to play football again and to finish with the chemotherapy.

My last treatment was not unlike all the others, except that subsequent visits would be for followup tests and check-ups and not the five-day cycle of drug injections. Tumor activity had decreased steadily during the previous two years, and by November 1975, Dr. Ruppenthal and Dr. Perlin were ready to call it quits with the chemo. It had been an experimental program, with no real predetermined timetable, and statistically it was surprising that not only was I still alive but also that I was better.

There is always hope for a cure, regardless of unfavorable medical opinion, and I, and I alone, was the one who controlled how I would handle my recovery program. It is the same for any cancer patient. I was thankful that the chemotherapy and radiation had worked. I was willing to pay any price so that they were effective, but had the therapy failed to arrest the disease I would still have worked toward accomplishing my goals. I could die before reaching them, but the effort was all part of my recovery. I'd experienced both the good and the bad of cancer, noting the exhilaration of an improved tumor marker and the resignation of unfavorable test results.

"Don't you feel lucky?" I was asked by many people. Not really. You determine your own future preparing to meet opportunity and, besides, I had made a request to God. I was fortunate, not lucky, and I knew the disease could kill me—indeed, I watched it kill others, but it seemed to be such a waste of life to concentrate on the negative result.

My last night recovering from the chemotherapy was long, marked by nausea and vomit, but by daybreak I felt much better, better than I'd ever felt right after the therapy. I was still weak, but the euphoria at the conclusion of the chemotherapy masked the sickness I hated. Carol Smith picked me up at the hospital, and Phil Nelson was already at her house for a champagne breakfast celebration. I was ready to get back to devoting maximum effort toward football, no longer interrupted by the therapy. Chemo was finished—another goal accomplished.

Carol took a circuitous route back to her house at 36 Upshur Road. Almost two years since the nightfall when I had collapsed on the second-floor landing there.

She drove me to Bancroft afterwards, but passing the chapel I said, "Carol, please stop. Let me out here. Go on ahead. I'll be here for a few minutes. I can walk back from here."

I knew she understood, and as she drove off and I walked up the chapel steps, I felt a sense of deep inner peace.

I'd never been particularly religious, but I tried to believe and act in good conscience, perhaps because of the solid upbringing my parents gave me and the love of all my family. It was with a sense of gratitude that I went inside the chapel, and I remembered an earlier prayer offered from my Bethesda hospital bed. I was alone in the chapel and walked up the center aisle to kneel in the front row pew, the Tiffany window above and behind the altar uniquely colorful. Special hues graced the figure of Christ walking upon the waters. The words inscribed in marble above the stained glass were, on this day, meant especially for me: "Eternal Father strong to save."

I spent a few moments in quiet reflection. I'd asked God for his help, and there had been so many kind people and guided circumstances—Earle and Carol Smith, George and Sandra Welsh, Bruce and Letty Ruppenthal, Admiral Mack, Admiral McKee—the list is long. How was it that such people happened to have crossed my path at the same time? I was humbled by the experience and talked to God, yet it was not easy to explain or rationalize. I was a part of his plan, as everybody is. I read part of a small missalette that was in the pew and continued thinking, my concentration interrupted by a tour group that came forth noisily from the back of the chapel. I thought to myself, You know, not one of those people knows what I am doing here, and not one can comprehend just how close my partner—God—and I have been.

I stood up after the group left and walked close to the altar, staring at Jesus set in stained glass, looking at him for what must have been several minutes, feeling closer and closer, even imagining God nodding at me again. What satisfaction I felt! "Thank you," I said out loud. I turned around slowly and walked back down the aisle. The closer I got to the exit, the faster my pace became, and when I opened the doors the sky was a deep blue and the sun remarkably bright—no more chemo, no more interruptions, no more vomiting and fever. I could get back into shape—there was no looking back. "Thank you, God," I said again, closing the doors behind me. I was free.

There was a lot of work left to be done. The therapy had run roughshod over my conditioning. I wasn't as fast, as big, or as quick as I'd been before the Michigan game of 1973. I had to stop and rest three times walking up the stairs to Coach Welsh's office when I went to ask permission to come out for football practice in the spring of 1976. I kept after it, trying to lift a little more each day and run a little farther. Coach Welsh's biggest concern was that I could get hurt, but after he and Coach Bresnahan checked with Dr. Ruppenthal, they told me I'd be issued gear in March.

I met Father Tom Donaher that spring while getting a haircut, overhearing a conversation from the chair next to me. "I'm supposed to start this drug treatment, this, ah, chemotherapy, sometime this weekend. I've heard a lot of things about that stuff. I wonder what it's like."

The word *chemotherapy* woke me up. Somebody was talking about it to one of the barbers.

"Ah, wait a second," I said to my own barber, and sat straight up, pushing the turn lever of my chair to swivel and face the person who was talking.

"Let me tell you about chemotherapy," I said, not to a midshipman but to an older, handsome, fortyish, gray-haired man, thin, of average height, who smiled at me with an inquisitive look.

"Yes?" he said.

"Tom Harper," I replied as we reached over and shook hands between the barbers.

"Midshipman Harper," I said again, remembering I was

addressing an officer I hadn't seen before. I didn't want to tell him that he'd puke his guts out, that he could lose all that good-looking hair, that his handsome face could be run over by acne, or that his hands would look funny, all yellow. I skirted the issue of chemo, and we talked a little about radiation therapy. I sympathized with him when he told me he had had a kidney failure, heart attack, and other problems before cancer.

He smiled again, seeming very content as his barber made a couple of touchup snips and loosened the striped sheet that covered his clothes. He looked at me and said, "I'm sorry. I forgot to introduce myself. Tom Donaher."

I looked over and saw his uniform blouse hanging by the door, a small gold-threaded cross sewn on the sleeve.

"Father Tom Donaher," he said, standing up and extending his hand.

"Tom, I'd like to talk with you some more."

"Yes, Father, I'm in the 17th Company."

"It was a pleasure to meet you, Tom. I've heard a lot about you. Looks like you took care of cancer."

"And you will too, Father."

Spring ball finally arrived, and I tried to reinforce my confidence by talking about it with my roommate and Commander Fellowes. It was hard to do what I'd done so easily before. I could go three plays at a high energy level, but anything after that hurt. My lungs were still only half full. I kept a small diary for a few days, relaxing after practice by sitting quietly in my room and writing a few notes on my small memo pad.

> DAY 1
> 22 March
> Practice was relatively easy—played at fifth string and alternated with fourth string every other play or so. I think it was easy because of the time between plays. I did make a few mistakes running pass patterns. Tranquil jumped on me for it. Must memorize my plays—hardest part of the practice was the 10 by 40s at the end—I felt like my legs were going to fall off. Welsh asked me how I was feeling and said that I didn't have to run

the sprints. I told him I'd do them slow, but *I did them*. Spaz gave me the thumbs up, and Bres asked me how I did. Felt great to put on pads, and I feel a lot more a part of the team. I hope I'm not embarrassing them with my conditioning at the end of practice. Felt good to go back and find it hard to believe—I know I can do it. I have to do it.

I felt like I'd never left. My pads were comfortable, and my helmet was snug. Had it really been two years? Was this the beginning of my junior season? Remember those great games against Michigan, Pitt, Notre Dame, and Army? What games? But then the huddle would break, and I wouldn't know what the play was.

DAY 2
23 March
Felt good today—a little more hitting and faster pace. Still a pain to play fifth team—don't like holding dummies. Thud [a scrimmage of about five plays] was fun, and I think I'm getting the hang of things. 10 by 40s at the end of practice—not as hard as yesterday. Made one nice catch but felt like it took me a year to get to the ball. Welsh asked me how I was holding up—told him I was having fun—which I am—I really enjoy it—feel a part of the team. Tomorrow we're supposed to do a lot of hitting. We'll see. Doc Rupp was at the beginning of practice. Good to see him.

I felt awkward, uncoordinated, embarrassed, and though I still had the hands, my reaction was way off, my reflexes were bad, and I was dying after two sprints. I reminded myself of the fat guys in high school who were always last.

"You don't have to run these sprints, Tom," Coach Welsh told me.

"I know, Coach, but I'll run them."

Was he trying to tell me I was embarrassing the team?

DAY 3
24 March
Felt good today—received my first good solid hit—Sandy Jones (WR) ran wrong pattern which ran three guys into me as I was going for the ball—hurt like hell—but I loved it—got some cramps today during thud, once while at the line of scrimmage. Commander Smith and Carol were there, but I didn't see them.

Went head-on with Julius—he beat me—won't happen again.
Getting tired of standing around. I'm better than Vogel.

I felt worse after practice when I overheard a plebe player
say to another, "Who's 88? Did they recruit him? He's terrible!
He's always last in the pass drills and keeps bending over to
catch his breath. He's really in bad shape."

I didn't feel like writing for a few days but then I picked
up.

DAY 7
27 March
First scrimmage—I wasn't very good. Played about 15–20 plays
overall. Tended to get tired after four consecutive plays. Didn't
block well and ran patterns very sloppy. During pass scrimmage
ran the wrong patterns and dropped the ball. But did manage to
catch one pass—should have been a TD but too tired to really
put any moves or speed on the defensive back. It's very embarrassing to be so bad—awfully frustrating. I hope the coaches
won't give up any confidence they might have in me. Must keep
trying. I do feel a lot better than a week ago. Still having a lot of
fun and enjoy being part of the team.

The best part of practice was the pass drills, running
routes against a loose defense, where I arranged it so that I
was rested every time it was my turn, telling guys ahead of
me to go ahead of me until I was ready. It was hard to adjust
to not being good, especially when a freshman would knock
me down. I waited a few days before I wrote again.

LAST DAY
12 April
I've missed a few days of writing—lazy, I guess—anyway, today was the last day of practice until after Spring Break. Felt
good today—even though I dropped a pass and misread a
block. We've had two more scrimmages—didn't play very
much, only a couple of series. Today was the first day they let
me in on thud—every other one. Before I was standing around
the last 45 minutes of practice doing nothing—so I asked Spaz
to let me in some more. He did, and I appreciated it. I did feel a
little quicker today, but I have a long way to go. Who knows?
Also, last Saturday (April 10), I was told I might be nominated
for a courage award from the American Cancer Society. I would

like to win that—would be most satisfying and gratifying.
Would also give me a little publicity, which would help other
people who might have cancer. They could relate to my cancer
and follow in my footsteps. Who knows? Will attempt to run
and lift over Spring Break, and be ready for the Blue–Gold
game. Then it's work on grades—grades are bad but not my
number one priority right now.

I wasn't in many scrimmages during spring ball, and
ended up finally on the fourth team. I remember one play
distinctly—the same play I ran during practice almost three
years earlier as a blue chip plebe, when I'd wiped out Chet
Moeller, our All-American safety. I tried it again, doing it the
same way, but I couldn't make the block, my opponent toss-
ing me aside to make the tackle. I was hit hard on
a pass route the very next play, fumbling, and before hitting the ground I thought to myself, I never would have
dropped the ball before.

I played every other play during the Blue–Gold game for
the Gold team offense, bringing in the signals, running
routes, blocking, and catching a couple of passes. I did well
for three downs, but there simply was not enough air to
breathe. I completed a pass route on one play, across the field
from the direction of the toss, and saw a player about my
height make a spectacular leaping catch before falling out of
bounds. Players on the sidelines were excited, and I heard
one of them shout, "Who made that catch? Was that Harper?"
I wanted it to be, and I backed off from the group, slowly
shaking my head that it wasn't.
I finished the Blue–Gold scrimmage as the third team
tight end. Coach Welsh never thought I'd really come back for
spring ball, and he had been justly apprehensive about it. I
had thought about football every day since September 28,
1973, and I knew that some day, some way, I would play
again. I thought about football while lying naked in my own
vomit at Bethesda. I thought about football lying alone in that
dismal radiation chamber. I thought about football as the
chemo with its sickening smell drained into my body.
I'd entered, however, into a tougher contest than football

when I was diagnosed with testicular cancer. Never had I been on such an emotional roller coaster, never had I been exposed to so many different attitudes about life and dying. Life is emotion, good or bad, and I'd experienced at a relatively early age the extremes of it, from depressing anguish to overwhelming joy. I'd been an ego-conscious midshipman football player who used that ego to survive, and I didn't care what other people said, or so I told myself.

If testicular cancer was going to kill me, it would have to interrupt my life. I wasn't going to let it stop me from working to reach my goals. I saw people give in to disease, and it was almost a guarantee that they would die. They had lost their appreciation for life. But I also witnessed the better side, and those people who did the best they could with what they had, whether they lived or died, were successful, and certainly contributed to the quality of my life. I was a beneficiary of unprecedented circumstances at the Naval Academy, and my diagnosis, recovery, and exposure to so many caring people was a window on positive emotion. One of the nurses told me, after my last chemotherapy treatment, "Well, you can start to live a normal life now."

I just looked at her and replied, "I have always led a normal life."

CHAPTER TWELVE

I hitchhiked from Quantico, Virginia, to Annapolis on the first Saturday of second class summer, arriving at 36 Upshur Road promptly at 8:00 P.M. Everyone was seated, waiting for me on the living room couch.

"Thanks for waiting for me," I began, standing in the center of the room. "I just wanted to tell you all thank you for everything . . . I love you."

I gave Jennifer and Shannon stuffed animals, a model ship to Earle Jr., and handed Carol and Commander Smith separate envelopes with money orders enclosed. They both looked puzzled, and Commander Smith said, "Tom, what is this for? You shouldn't do this."

"Commander Smith, please, no questions. I wanted to get you both a present, but couldn't decide, so you and Carol pick out your own wardrobe. Carol, that money order is good only for the shop that's on it. Sandra told me about it. It's a neat place. Commander Smith, you must promise you'll use it only for a sports jacket."

I pointed to the envelope in his hand, and then Earle stood up and we hugged each other and I embraced Carol and all the kids.

They gave me a ride back to the beltway in the morning, offering to drive me all the way back to Quantico.

"Here we are," I said, as we passed a green, reflective highway sign that pointed Richmond to the south, and Commander Smith drove over to the shoulder of the road and stopped.

"I can make it from here."

"Are you sure, Tom? We don't mind bringing you on in," Commander Smith replied, turning around from behind the steering wheel.

"You've gone out of your way already. It's no problem, really."

I opened the side door and got out. It was not easy to say goodbye. The kids would grow up and leave for school somewhere, and the Smiths' new duty station, Pearl Harbor, was on the other side of the world. I can still see the kids' melancholy faces as we said goodbye, Commander Smith and Carol taking a part of me with them when they drove away.

Second class summer was interesting exposure to the Marine Corps in Virginia, submarines at New London, Connecticut, ships at Newport, Rhode Island, and Navy Air at Pensacola, Florida. The week-long Marine indoctrination in Quantico was relatively loose and marked by recent graduates drinking beer and eating potato chips with us on the Bachelor Officers' Quarters quarterdeck, as they talked about how great the Corps was. We were flown out by helicopters to training fields some ten miles from the main facilities. All flights were grounded one day, forcing us to march back, the grunts in our group having the keen desire to run with rifles at high port.

I dropped further and further back from the platoon, exhorted for over a mile by a new second lieutenant to "C'mon, c'mon, keep up, keep up!" He finally left me alone, coming up later to apologize once he was made aware of my restricted pulmonary function. Things like that were something I had to learn to live with.

The Newport BOQ was considerably more habitable, the accommodations there a welcome improvement from the boondocks of Quantico. New London was the same, and although I couldn't go aboard the submarines or fly in jet aircraft as we finished summer training in Pensacola, the exposure to the Navy outside of Bancroft was a rewarding experience. I managed a helicopter ride over the Gulf Coast beaches, the pilot letting me fly some from the right seat, where I promptly threw up. I was thankful it was from air sickness, though, and not those nauseating drugs.

Spring football had been fun, but I was out of my league and, while at home during summer leave, I realized my time as a football player was over. I enjoyed workouts back at Oceana as a former player who went on to college football, but when I tried the mile under six minutes and thirty seconds with the high school players, I struggled to finish. The schoolboy halfbacks were quicker and hard to keep up with, much less defense. I'd hinted before about something like this only to Commander Fellowes.

"I don't have the endurance anymore," I'd told him, those words coming back as I tried to compete on the playing fields of Pacifica, California. I was improving with the breathing tests, telling the Annapolis corpsmen, "One of these days, I'm going to pop it," referring to the pulmonary machine bag, but my exhale–inhale capacity was still not much more than half that of an average person.

I'd caught a perfect pass in the Blue–Gold game, right over the middle, and there was one defensive back between me and the end zone, 40 yards away, but I ran right toward him with my head down. He didn't tackle me—I tackled myself into him because I was too tired to make any moves and run any further. I remembered thinking then, as we both fell in a heap to the turf, that if this was three years ago, this guy wouldn't have had a chance; I would have scored. I walked back to the huddle, and Coach Spaz looked quizzical, raising his eyebrows and saying, "That should have been a touchdown."

"I know . . . tired," I responded with a sign, the coach's look saying, "Tom, maybe one day you were good, but not now. Sorry."

I had played football again, which was a goal, but deep down I realized I was no longer a good player. Cancer had taken away more than I realized. I telephoned the Welshes from home, and after talking with Sandra I asked to speak with George, who, aware of my frustration, said, "Tom, you don't have to prove anything to us. The great thing is that you wanted to come out and play again. You were here the first day and every day, in pads, you did everything, you hit people. You made people believe."

I didn't know what to answer, and when Coach Welsh invited me to join the team as a coach for summer practice, I accepted. Athletic tasks that were once easy and almost second nature to me were now very difficult, and I was thinking, more than reacting, on the football field.

I continued lifting weights and ran a little further each day. We had some new plebe linemen with excellent potential, and I helped them progress with weight training and speed drills. Cancer left me without the conditioning to be a starting tight end, but I was a part of the Navy football team from the day I took the oath of a midshipman to the day I graduated.

Dr. Ruppenthal's checkups and examinations became as much a part of my day as glazed doughnuts for breakfast. I enjoyed a 4N morning (four straight classes) and superburgers for lunch, followed by the enjoyment of rack time, a youngster afternoon of no classes. You could lower the blinds, shut the door, sleep in the artificial darkness, and make up for late-hour bull sessions. The Academy hospital and Bethesda kept a close watch on me, and my checkups were always good. Soon the doctors were able to pronounce a complete remission, but there was still some question about whether or not I would receive a commission.

It was a busy second class year—a constant mix of study, class, and the myriad of other extracurricular activities. I'd take my mind off the book in front of me during breaks from analyzing a particularly tough subject, to think about what I'd really learned.

I'd always feel better after lifting weights and thus reacted to chemo better; when I scored well on a test, I did well with the therapy. It wasn't an altogether dissatisfying experience— at times, it was more like a game, and I concentrated on doing only those things that would help me. I was certainly aware of the seriousness of cancer, but I never wanted it to affect my life style. I saw people with similar afflictions sometimes look the other way and, with cancer, they tend to think of movies and TV shows which, though applauding courage, contribute to the fear of cancer and the idea of certain defeat. This does nothing for those who want to live. I want to help people think of something else—someone who lived. It wasn't Tom Harper that was important, but the concept of life, and though some will comment that I was young and overly optimistic, the only way anyone should approach cancer is with the will to win. Dr. Ruppenthal told my father I had not been cured by medicine alone. While positive emotion cannot always break the association between cancer and dying, whatever therapy is applied without a positive attitude is only made more difficult. My own treatment had been a series of choices and decisions. If I had let myself be influenced to an excessive extent by fault-finders, I could easily have come to dwell on dying.

Doctors and nurses are involved with innumerable life and death situations, some of them coping by blocking out their own emotions. A human being can only handle so much, and the gradual buildup of pressure can cause anybody to deny their own feelings, making it hard to help others effectively. I never observed any such difficulty with Dr. Perlin or Dr. Ruppenthal and can only classify their efforts as splendid. Friends were always around to take my mind off the chemotherapy and cancer, reinforcing the feeling that, to them, I was always the same. My cancer had been exactly that—my cancer—and I did not need to share it but wanted certainly the sustenance and camaraderie of those close to me.

I was invited to speak at the national convention of the volunteers of the American Cancer Society in Atlanta during the winter. I had not been approached by the ACS during the course of my therapy, nor did I know much about the organization other than its nameplate on literature and the several celebrities who gave their name to the ACS cause. I felt honored and began reciting lines walking back from class, practicing speaking gestures while working out, and going over in my mind what I'd said to the football team after my last chemo treatment:

> As most of you know, I had my last chemotherapy treatment last Saturday, and . . . ah . . . I asked Coach Welsh to let me talk to you. I just want to say thanks. There were many times when I came into the locker room, and you guys would always ask me how I was doing. Commander Smith used to tell me how all you guys asked about me. After each chemo, somebody would always ask me how I was doing, and somebody would always help me with my workouts. I want to thank you for your support for the past three years. Without you, I may not have been here today. Some of you are new, and a lot of players have graduated, but your support kept me going. I can never tell you just how big a help you've been. I'm looking forward to coming back out, and I just wanted to say . . . thank you for helping me be here.

What would I tell this new audience? That you had to get sick to cure a cancer? That the side effects were bad? That the fear of pain is sometimes worse than the fear of death? What is the prime ingredient of success? That you needed faith, belief, and trust in God? Admiral McKee drilled into us that professionals were people who made a habit, in order to accomplish a goal, of doing the things they didn't like to do, as well or better than the things they preferred. Would I tell them that?

I was nervous in Atlanta, my butterflies dancing that night with stage fright, but I was glad to do something for the many volunteers there. Leif Erickson, the distinguished actor, made an eloquent introduction, and I followed with these short remarks:

> Three years ago, when my doctors told me I had a malignant tumor and a spreading disease and might not live much longer, I suffered a blow that knocked me down; but I didn't stay down, and that is what is important . . . to bounce back. I lost all my hair, lost over 50 pounds, had a severe complexion problem, and even had trouble walking up three flights of stairs. During this time, I discovered the great healing power of work.

> If you are lonely, work! If you are worried or fearful, work! If you are discouraged or defeated, work! Work is the key! I'm not playing football anymore but another game that we all learn to play—a game called life. Cancer gave me lessons of what life is all about—humility, faith, and courage. When you play sports, you learn to win and you learn to lose. There's a difference between a good loser and learning how to lose. I was never a good loser, but losing teaches you something. It teaches you to have hope and accept a challenge . . .

I paused momentarily, my nervousness subsiding as I finished by paraphrasing a quote:

> Challenge is the core and mainspring of human activity. If there's a mountain, we climb it. If there's an ocean, we cross it. If there's a wrong, we right it. And finally, for you members of the American Cancer Society and hardworking volunteers, if there's a disease, we cure it."

I was asked to speak again, and in the ensuing months I met several celebrities, politicians, film stars, and media personalities. I just hoped my speeches helped somebody realize that cancer is not always incurable.

The class of 1977 graduated in June, and I was the first to salute Phil Nelson, who repaid me with the traditional sum of one dollar. We both wondered when we'd see each other again, since some guys graduate and don't see one another for five, ten, 15 years, or longer. Phil was going Navy Air, and I was traveling across the country on behalf of the ACS, but it seemed inevitable that we'd cross paths. We talked often on the telephone during my final year, the main point of conversation being what I'd do if I wasn't offered a commission. The commission was the official stamp of approval and served to extinguish any negative connotation between my name and cancer.

I departed for first class summer cruise on the USS *Independence* with my grades finally at an acceptable level, considering the number of speeches I'd made all over the country. The *Independence* had a motivated crew, and I spent more than a month in the Mediterranean. I enjoyed watching the flight operations from the carrier deck, and I understood then why my older brother and most of my friends wanted to fly. If I was commissioned, it would be in the Supply Corps, and so I volunteered to work in the supply department on board, my motivation enhanced by the opportunity to contribute something, even if I was part of the *Independence* for just a short period of time. I'd been through with the chemo for more than a year, though shots of chest pain and aching lungs would frequently remind me of it, and I couldn't make it up past the captain's deck of the aircraft carrier's tower. But I was able to walk the flight deck and maneuver in, out, and around most of the ship's various passageways and ladders with much improved dexterity.

I stopped by Father Donaher's quarters after cruise, intending to say hello before leaving for California, but he wasn't home. Father Donaher had devoted his Easter sermon to talk about me, and though I wasn't there to hear it, I wanted to thank him. Father Donaher had been undergoing regular treatments, but his body wasn't adapting to the rigors of therapy, and I learned at home in August that he'd died. I spoke to the congregation at the chapel after the Brigade returned, about his stature as a priest, a man, and a cancer patient who never complained. I never imagined I'd be speaking from a church pulpit about anybody, but Father Donaher had spoken highly of me, and I wanted to talk about this good man:

> Good morning. This morning I am going to share with you the companionship I was fortunate to have with Father Donaher. He told me once that we cannot expect to live always on a smooth and even plane. We all face problems, worries, and fears. We all have our setbacks, our sorrows, and our misfortunes. They are part of the substance of living, and none of us can escape them. Father Donaher was faced with sorrow, pain, and fear. But through it all, he endured and calmly went on. He endured nauseating chemotherapy treatments, the pain of radiation, and all the fears of cancer. I, too, have had cancer. I have gone through over two years of chemotherapy treatments and one year of radiation, together with the fear of dying. After I

met Father Donaher, he became a special strength for me. The way he handled his disease was a definition of everything I had fought for. When I went through radiation treatments, it was common for me to hear people speaking of death. When they were told they had cancer, they would ask, "When will I die?" but Father Donaher had to say, not "When will I die?" but "How much longer do I have to live?" Father Donaher did the best he could with what he had. He knew that it is not what you have lost, but what you have left that counts. We both understood together what it means to have cancer. We both helped each other. This little verse by William Merkel best explains our friendship: "I am going your way, so let us go hand in hand. You help me, and I will help you. We shall not be here very long, for soon death will come rock us all to sleep. Let us help one another while we may." His special strength became my support. The message I received from Father Donaher is best understood by quoting Robert Louis Stevenson: "Keep your fears to yourself, but you must share your courage with others."

First class year was my final and most responsible year as a midshipman. Five years had been devoted to the position and I was anxious to start from the best possible advantage. The plebe football players I'd helped coach the previous season were now third class, bigger and stronger than the year before, and it was gratifying to see them perform at a more capable level.

I was on the plebe detail for a portion of the summer, and before starting my regime I brought my whole squad into the company head at 0300, commissioning them to compose a "Harper Squad Song," to be conducted and sung in the mess hall during meals. Twelpin would have been appalled.

The Seventh Wing Players, an anonymous group of mids, often performed in the parking lot of our wing, to mock Academy protocol with varying degrees of obscenity. Those desiring to participate had to satisfy the entrance requirement of physically kidnapping an unsuspecting mid, stripping him naked, and tying him to a chair. The victim would be deposited in the parking lot, to be covered by shaving cream, water from the overlooking windows, and layers of verbal abuse. Humor was an absolute requirement.

The Army–Navy game that year attracted the largest television audience of the college football season, marked unfortunately by Army's victory after the ball slipped out of the grasp of a Navy receiver on the Cadets' goal line, with only seconds remaining on the clock. I was in the coaches' box helping to spot plays and couldn't believe it, hating to lose to Army after four consecutive wins.

I still ran a mile for every year since my biopsy, every September 28, and completed a four-mile run during the fall of first class year. Several people expressed concern about my chances of recurrence, but my chances of having it again are no greater than anyone else's.

I spent Easter break in Pensacola, Florida, where Phil Nelson and Tom Hutchinson were in flight training, and we spent hours water skiing. I got food poisoning from one of the finer establishments on Pensacola's main drag, which scared me, since I felt just as sick as I had during the chemotherapy. Although I recovered in three days, everyone, including me, feared a relapse.

Anyone with cancer has to learn to live with things like this, which emphasizes the value of regular checkups and a good exercise program. This proved to me that cancer recovery is not over once the actual treatment is stopped.

A University of Maryland fraternity staged a 72-hour dance marathon for the benefit of the American Cancer Society in November. It was an annual tradition in memory of a fraternity member who'd died with the disease, and I was invited to speak.

The benefit began with a story of a girl dying of cancer—a short movie was shown about her courageous background and her desire to share everything with everybody, but after the first few minutes of the film, I blocked it out of my mind. The script emphasized death—not only the emotional issue of the death of a pretty girl, but more importantly the dramatization of a strong opinion that she was going to die.

The lights in the auditorium stayed dark for a few minutes after the film, the whole place as quiet as an empty church, and then a single shaft of light came out from the upper levels of the back of the building to highlight the master of ceremonies, who stood up and said, "You've all seen the movie. But there is a victory over cancer. Tonight, we have with us a 23-year-old Naval Academy midshipman who was diagnosed with cancer in 1973 and given three months to live. He has beaten the disease, and today, ladies and gentlemen, he is quite alive. Ladies and gentlemen, Tom Harper."

The spotlight shifted directly to me before I could stand. Jesus Christ, I thought to myself, walking to the podium in front of which was a sea of faces, boxed in on all sides by large signs that glowed "Dance Against Cancer" from the shadows. What am I going to say to these people after a film like that?

> I love music, and I love to dance . . . I learned a lot about humility, I learned a lot about faith, I learned a lot about courage, and, most importantly, I learned a lot about people. I learned that there are people who care, people like yourselves who are willing to work for worthy causes. You cannot pursue happiness and catch it. Happiness comes upon you unaware while you are helping others. I am cured of cancer, half because I was game to take a wicked amount of punishment along the way and half because there were an awful lot of people who cared enough to help. It was a bewildering, challenging, and exhausting experience. But if it means that my experience awakens people to the fact that cancer can be beaten with dedication and hard work, then my recovery memories are certainly less painful. I hope by meeting with you tonight you have seen that there is victory over cancer. We've seen a tragic movie, but we must learn by laughter as well as by tears. The motto for tonight, "Dance against Cancer," is beautiful. You are finding happiness by working for a worthy cause. Your happiness comes from putting your hearts in your work and doing it with joy and enthusiasm.

I thanked them for their efforts in staging such an extravaganza but cannot recall, even immediately after finishing, the rest of what I said. The film had overshadowed any comments I could make. There was a tremendous electricity to the crowd, but my reaction to the movie had been a mirror of my own emotions at Bethesda.

Commander Fellowes had arranged, unbeknownst to me, to have word get back to the American Cancer Society's New York headquarters about a Naval Academy midshipman and his fight against cancer. The ACS looks every year for a story of a traumatic experience that proves favorable, to demonstrate that cancer doesn't always kill you. The Academy had kept me enrolled in the face of negative medical evidence, saying, in effect, that cancer is not incurable and doesn't have to totally dominate your life.

Previous awards, always signed and presented by the president of the United States, had gone to such notables as Mike Finamore, a leukemia patient; Jack Pardee, professional football player and coach; Gene Litler, a golfer; singers Margaret Piazza and Minnie Ripperton; actor William Gargan; and even a cadet from West Point, Robert Johnson. I was selected to receive the 1978 ACS Courage Award. I was thrilled to be recognized and honored to follow in the footsteps of earlier recipients.

The ACS flew my parents out for the presentation at the White House. Everybody in my family sent telegrams to Mom and Dad's hotel room in Washington and to the superintendent's house at the Academy, where Admiral McKee had invited Mom and Dad to spend the night before the presentation.

The messages read:

Congrats. You've earned this.
So very, very proud.
Courage takes faith, so keep the faith, baby.
Much love, Susie and Mike.

You're in DC
To see JC
With Mom and Pops
You rise to the top
Your claim to fame
Will bring us no shame
But we can say we knew you when . . .
Congratulations, Jackie.

Congratulations from Texas on two points:

1. Pop's speedy recovery.
2. Tom's long overdue recognition.
Randy, Rose, Stella, and Dorothy send their best.

Dear Tom, we rejoice with you today as the president of the
United States bestows upon you the National Courage Award of
the American Cancer Society. We wish we could be with you in
the White House as you receive this great honor.
With love, Grandfather and Uncle Bill.

My younger sisters, Sally and Theresa, topped everything
off by bringing back a childhood nickname, the telex from San
Francisco proclaiming:

Tom the Bomb, you've really exploded this time!

I had an extra instruction literature class the morning of
the presentation but excused myself early, saying to the prof,
"I've got to go meet the president."

"Sure you do, Harper," he replied, and I couldn't help
but grin as I left Mahan Hall to meet my parents at the Capitol
Hilton.

We met Admiral McKee there and Marvella Bayh, the
wife of the senator from Indiana and a courageous cancer patient herself. We were driven by limousine to the White
House, where we were shown to the Roosevelt Room. I was
happy Marvella was there, as she had listened to several of
my speeches and we'd often talked afterwards. She had a cancer far more advanced than mine, but she had resolved to get
the most out of each and every day.

Rosalyn Carter came into the room, accompanied by
some Japanese dignitaries, and was shortly followed by her
press secretary, who informed us that the president was ready
to see us.

Mom entered the Oval Office first, and I followed, then
Dad and the rest of the entourage came in.

"Mr. President, Dorothy Harper," Mom said, stepping
aside as the president smiled in return. Someone said, "Mr.
President, Midshipman Tom Harper."

The ceremony was a touching event, if only to see my

parents in the company of the president of the United States. Everyone listened attentively as President Carter spoke and presented the award. I kept my comments brief, and no sooner did it seem we entered the White House than I was standing in the East Wing with my parents, the three of us alone, waiting for our limousine.

"I can't believe I'm doing this," Mom said, "standing here in the White House, waving goodbye to everyone."

Dad and I joined in her laughter.

Filming the 1978 ACS inspirational film took five days. The mechanics of the Tapper production were fascinating, and they took shots of my workouts as I ran around the track or up the stadium steps, and included scenes with Dr. Ruppenthal, the Welshes, and Chris Picchi, who recounted the recovery room awakening almost five years before. The crew would return for the graduation scenes, the atmosphere of cameras, dialogue, and lights adding to the excitement of finishing six years of effort. I found it hard to believe I was getting all of this attention.

The Academy made a video presentation of my recovery and my former seapower prof, Commander Gordie Petersen, wrote an article with Ellen Ternes of the Academy's Public Affairs Office, entitled "One Step at a Time," which appeared in the alumni magazine and several Navy publications worldwide. Newspapers across the country printed articles about the ACS award, and all the while I still wasn't sure I'd reach my goal of receiving a commission.

The ACS award was special, the film was nice, the attention and celebrity status, even my appearance on the *Today Show*, were great, but without receiving final approval in the form of "Ensign, USN," everything was incomplete. Admiral McKee, however, gave me his full support, and the final Medical Board read:

> At this time, Midshipman Harper has no signs of recurrent disease. It is most likely that he has been cured of his disease. Although it has gradually improved over the last two years, his pulmonary function has been partially compromised as a result of radiation therapy and chemotherapy. Nevertheless, he is con-

sidered completely fit for commissioning in the Staff Corps and/
or restricted line of duty limited to the shore establishment. He
should continue to have periodic reevaluations at six-month intervals."

I did not hear anything affirmative until the morning of graduation.

June Week arrived quicker than expected, my parents,
brothers, and sisters arriving from a variety of states to share
in the many festivities. Everyone had gone to considerable ex-
pense and effort to be together, and even the hectic schedule
could not change the commitment I had to share the best moments with my family.

Graduation was always so far away, and yet the time now
was so short. The night before graduation, all of my family,
along with Phil Nelson's parents, assembled at the Library, a
pleasant, cozy Annapolis restaurant. We spent the evening in
good company, with food and spirits, trading stories and
jokes back and forth, our laughter and cheer filling the establishment with noise and the enjoyment of a happy family reunion.

It's real. My presence is why I wanted to do this book,
and I thought about that as I looked that night around the
table, admiring the happy faces of those who had traveled so
far to share my graduation. Dad toasted Mary Beth on behalf
of both of us, everyone joining in to second the accolade.

I went through so much just to graduate and wanted to
be part of what the Naval Academy stands for. Without the
foundation provided by the people who dined with me at the
Library and the contribution of my Academy family, I would
not have had the tools to survive and compete with cancer on
my own terms.

Dad rose to stand at the head of the table, getting our
attention by tapping his glass of red wine with the point of a
silver dinner knife. He held out the goblet, the liquid bathed in
candle reflections and the soft light returned from the table
setting, and Mom, Mary Beth, Randy, Jackie, Susie, Sally,
Theresa, Richard, and the Nelsons all stood up.

Dad tipped his glass toward me, and more than just past

recollections masked the tears I hid behind my smiling face. The sense of accomplishment was immense, and I knew I was starting a new chapter in my life, ably prepared by past experiences and a keenly developed sense of purpose. I was not a victim. I did what I set out to do, no better recognized than by the smiling faces of my family on a night forever in my memory.

"Tom," Dad said, "it is not without a sense of humor that we have gathered here this evening, but neither is it without a true feeling of love and admiration for what you have accomplished. We salute you, and all the people who made this night possible, and the fine school from which you are about to graduate."

CHAPTER THIRTEEN

I was one of the 938 first class midshipmen spending our last morning, June 7, 1978, in Bancroft Hall. The window blinds in my room were drawn to the top, inviting the scenery from the ground and water below to fill the panes of glass I had cleaned so often. The sky was slightly overcast, with a low-lying bucket of clouds darkening the Severn River, which emptied in the distance into the Chesapeake Bay. The spotted lacrosse field was directly below my window, and across the narrow asphalt of Santee Road sailing craft were moored, with names such as *Vigilant, Swift,* and *Lively.* Old Luce Hall was to the left of my view, and I thought of signal flags, Morse code, and plotting navigational charts as I watched seagulls glide in for a landing on top of the long building. They matched flight with the steady clanging of brass bells from the knockabouts underneath, a peaceful sound, never an interruption, and a lucid mixture passing through with calming regularity.

I glided over a sparkling floor that would no doubt get us past the final inspection. My roommate and I had gear astrew and tossed about, but that would be packed away shortly into cruise boxes filled with years of accumulated debris. The printing on my box read:

THOMAS J. HARPER
500589765
ENSIGN USN

It seemed to put a lid over the six years since I'd left home. The commission status from my medical board was to have

193

been forwarded from the Navy's Bureau of Personnel, and I reminded myself to walk down to the Midshipman Personnel office as soon as it opened. The package had been held up all week, and I didn't want any more undue delay.

My family rented a private Annapolis home for the June Week festivities, and for the first time in seven years we were all together, eight brothers and sisters. It was a pleasant reunion, especially for my parents, and I was the only midshipman with five beautiful dates—all my sisters accompanying me during the best week of my life.

I was sure everybody at the house was still asleep as I finished packing, but I was too psyched to try to sleep, especially after receiving a telegram from a high school friend, Steve Haskins, who was on duty overseas with the Marines. "Well, Tom, this is it," he wrote. "What you set out to do is now coming true."

Annapolis graduation is not a droning, black-gowned affair, but a special ceremony, a proud commencement, and an event thought of from the first days of plebe year. I felt deep satisfaction for myself, my family, and close friends, because many people would receive diplomas today, and though mine proclaimed Thomas Jackson Harper, many other names should have been transcribed with it. I hadn't gone through everything alone.

Our class stood outside the Navy–Marine Corps Memorial stadium for more than an hour before marching in, excitement and nervousness spreading throughout our ranks. I was wired for sound by an American Cancer Society film crew as we stood waiting, which was a welcome break in the monotony.

It was almost midday, the sky moist and overcast, the threat of rain bringing a cooling breeze that eased the humid Annapolis summer. It was like Worden Field parades when we entered the stadium, marching in to the assigned rows of seats on the playing field.

There were shadows over the letters that spell "Normandy" on the stadium's north parapet, and other names greeted this special afternoon—"Salerno," "Iwo Jima," "Leyte

Gulf," "Cape Glocester," "Chosen Reservoir"—lined with more accolades of battles set alongside the white concrete, evoking their own silent fascination of tradition and remembrance of sacrifice and the long ago dead. "Tarawa," "Coral Sea," "Midway," "Belleau Woods," "Eastern Solomons"—they seemed so far away, different, and set apart from the football that was usually played here.

The stadium is built in a high horseshoe, and cannon charges fired after a Navy score seem to roll along all the wood benches and metal seats in the stands. Anything that could be painted was covered in old blue and gold, and the inclined, cylindrical cement ramps to the upper decks appeared to be antiquated gun turrets, overlooking subtle testimony to naval tradition. Gate C to the north proclaimed the class of 1934's engraved words:

> They that go down to the sea in ships, that do business in great waters, they see the works of the Lord and the wonders of the deep.

There were extra precautions this year. The president of the United States was addressing the graduating class, and as it was a homecoming of sorts for him, the attendant media lent an air of organized confusion. It was an additional stimulant to the day I had devoted six years toward—a goal that kept me alive. These were my last moments as a midshipman, and by the time the evening sun faded behind the words of "Southern France," I would have proven not only to myself but to many others that faith and support predominate any unseen foe. It was a personal commitment, a vow not to lose, to keep going through radiation and toxic drug treatment, harassment and academic pressure, the feeling of others not really understanding. It was a goal that meant something different from just being able to say I graduated from the Naval Academy. I did it—with my body, my heart, and my soul, and with the many people who were an integral part of what the Naval Academy is all about.

We were flanked by Academy academic and military staff, and senior military and civilian officials were on the platform with the president, attended by the media with their cameras, microphones, and notebooks. A roving camera of the ACS film crew stayed near me, and one cameraman was close to my parents. I turned every now and then to look through the stands, knowing generally where everybody was sitting, but I was too far away to make out any faces. I was disappointed that the Smiths could not be there, but George and Sandra Welsh were seated with my family, as well as Bruce and Letty Ruppenthal, Jack Fellowes, and Phil Nelson. Admiral Mack, now retired, was with other dignitaries and officials on the graduation platform. I was especially pleased he was there.

The ceremony progressed smoothly. The president began his speech by noting that Admiral Nimitz had addressed the class of 1947 at their commencement but that Nimitz's comments were the last thing they cared about. All the president was thinking then was that he was graduating, getting married, and leaving USNA. The graduates' thoughts hadn't changed in 31 years as the president continued with a foreign policy address, excitement building as his remarks drew to a close. "Well, here we go," one soon-to-be ensign next to me kept saying.

The ceremony continued with acknowledgment of special achievements by various members of the graduating class, other comments by officials and dignitaries, but the superintendent's opening remarks stunned me.

"The personal courage of Tom Harper is a hallmark of this class," Vice Admiral McKee said. Since he wrote his own speeches, I knew he was speaking directly to me.

Top academic graduates were recognized and diplomas presented by name thoughout the 36 companies, accompanied by family applause scattered throughout the stadium. Company by company, the ceremony went, and soon the Lieutenant Commander usher we'd been watching reached our aisle—the 17th Company was being announced, and we all rose and took our place in line. I looked back momentarily at where my family was seated, and a few times as we moved along a name would ring out and the applause would be a little louder than usual. I thought about a lot of things as I approached the ramp—where the ACS film crew was, not falling down the ramp on my face, whether my plebes would stand as they had hinted they would, and that Admiral McKee would personally present my diploma. I found myself going back to football habits, rubbing my hands and rolling my shoulders as I straightened the uniform over my chest.

"Thomas J. Harper" was announced, the sound seeming to reverberate thoughout the stadium, and I walked up the ramp in as smart a military fashion as I could muster. There was silence for a brief second or two, then increasing, steady, rippling applause, becoming louder as I reached Admiral McKee. I looked the superintendent right in the eye and thanked him not only for the diploma but also for letting me stay at the Naval Academy. I felt his extra grip as we shook hands, and we lingered on the platform as he clasped my shoulder. I caught a glimpse of people moving and clapping, the class of 1978 standing up and applauding in a spontaneous ovation.

I clenched my fist in salute and was off the platform quickly and into a maze of handshakes and happy, shouted remarks, grabbing as many hands as I could on the way to my chair. I was in another world when I sat down, fighting back tears and telling myself, "Do not cry, do not cry, Tom Harper." I clenched my fists again and thanked the Lord, saying, "Thanks, God," my head bowed as I concentrated, "You did it, God. Without you . . . what else can I say?"

The president and first lady wanted to talk with me, and I was greeted by the Navy officer who, I recognized, always accompanied the president. "Go up the stairs, walk to the president, and introduce yourself," he said, and I did, offering my hand as the president and his wife stood up to ask how I was feeling.

"Great!" I replied, shaking Rosalyn Carter's hand and then the president's, thanking them for coming, and a group of people from that side of the podium applauded while I made my way back to my seat. It had been quite a moment—I was given a standing ovation, talked with the president, and people were still clapping. I stood by my chair, surrounded by happy faces and a cascade of white uniforms moving in every different direction. I was overwhelmed.

Dad's eyes were moist, the tears of joy from my mother's eyes matching the emotions of my five sisters, and Sandra Welsh and Letty Ruppenthal cried happily. Phil Nelson kept up with the applause, feeling goosebumps as his spine shivered, and Bruce Ruppenthal expressed the satisfaction they all felt with a wide smile. Coach Welsh, still wearing sunglasses on this overcast day, was sitting right behind my parents, and when I had gone up the ramp to meet Admiral McKee, he'd thought about all the earlier steps taken—the years of sickness and therapy, the catching up with academics, the workouts, my living with the Smith family. Everything today was capsulated together—all the review boards, the ups and downs, the turnback, being sick all the time, the anxiety over test results, the threat of recurrence, the loss of youth. I wished that Earle and Carol Smith and their kids could have been there.

The academic dean bestowed baccalaureate honors upon us and was followed by the chief of naval operations, who stood to lead us in the pledge of the oath of a naval officer. Our class president ran in leaps and bounds up the ramp to the microphone on the podium after the CNO finished, leaning into the mike and shouting, "Three cheers for those we leave behind! Hip, hip, hooray! Hip, hip, hooray! Hip, hip, hooray!" The final "hooray!" was only halfway out of our throats as we tossed our hats, all 938 of them hanging suspended in the air and then falling in a glorious mixture back to the playing field, bouncing off chairs and people, being stepped on and tossed away to little kids who ran out from the stands. I would meet my family by the goalposts in the west end zone. I had graduated, and I was commissioned!

The television networks, radio stations, journalists, newspaper photographers—everywhere I looked there was a camera or a microphone. People would stop and look, curious about the attention being given and the entourage we'd assembled. Mom had the gold-braided, black emblazoned ensign board for my left shoulder, and Sandra Welsh held the one for the right. It had happened!

Mom guided the board insignia under the thin straps on my uniform and snapped it into place, her touch a reminder that I was lucky to have such a woman to have brought me into this world. The fact that we both reached this moment brought me the sense of joy with which she is so amply endowed. She smiled with me, knowing what I felt as we shared our happiness together. Sandra attached the other shoulder board, whispering into my ear, "This is done with Carol Smith, also."

I had never seen my father speechless. We approached each other with our hands extended, looking eye to eye. No words can adequately say how much love I have for him. Dad, I thought, you just gave me the highest compliment. Thank you. He held back tears, masking emotion, but his pride and love were impossible to conceal, because this time not only the battle but the war had been won. Dad was recovering from a massive heart attack suffered a few months earlier, and I thanked God he was with us.

There was something indelibly written on this day, and we lingered on the football field, the moment a dream set deep in my soul, never to be forgotten. I remembered a major league baseball player telling of how he sat in the stands after he had set a record for RBIs in one game, staying until 3:00 or 4:00 A.M., not wanting to leave, enjoying what he had just done. When we walked out of the stadium, I took each step slowly, leaving an accomplishment behind and ready to enter the next phase of my life with renewed confidence and anticipation of the good things and people of the future.

The party started without me, while I went back to Bancroft to pick up records and gather personal belongings from 7242, my old room. I took one last look at the place, nodded my head as I clenched my fist, and left. I'd catered the party, and when I finally arrived, my family, friends, and guests were well into the celebration, plenty of champagne flowing, the spirit of good times ebbing from every happy face and well-wishing smile. I was greeted by my father, who raised his glass in a toast. I will never forget the words Dad said and, more importantly, how he said them, his arms strong and firm as he held his glass up high and toasted me in the clarity and purpose of voice I've always admired.

"Here's to five years successfully completed, and a goal sought for and accomplished. Tom, we love you, we're proud of you, and we thank you."

"Where's mine?" I replied, and raised the glass of champagne handed to me, saying, "Thank you all for coming. This celebration . . . is my thanks to you for your love and devotion in helping me accomplish the goal that we set out to do years ago. When they tell you that you have cancer, you can give up or you can fight. I chose to fight."

I paused slightly, looking at the group before me. "I thank God for the strength he gave to you to give to me."

EPILOGUE

The diagnosis and treatment of testicular cancer have come a long way since September 28, 1973. The chances of recovery, if diagnosis is made early enough, are excellent, and are far superior to those of ten years ago.

On June 15, 1983, Tom Harper was the proud father of a healthy baby boy. Tom, his wife Lynn, ten-year-old stepson, Billy, and Adam currently live in Virginia. Tom has a cured medical record and travels extensively as a professional speaker on motivation and health awareness.